Beat Hypertension Easily Using Nutrition

By

Lynne D M Noble

All rights reserved. No part of this publication may be reproduced, stored in a retrieval system or transmitted in any form or by any means, without prior permission in writing of the author Lynne D M Noble, or as expressly agreed by law, or under terms agreed with the appropriate reprographics right organisation.

You must not circulate this book in any other binding or cover and you must impose the same condition on any acquirer.

Independently published 2020

About the Author

Lynne Noble was born in 1953 in Huddersfield, West Yorkshire. From a very early age, Lynne showed an interest in nutrition and genetics avidly reading any books that she could get her hands on at the time.

Initially, Lynne studied orthopaedics but events led her to work with the elderly mentally infirm. Here, her interest in neurodegenerative disorders and pain syndromes developed.

Lynne undertook rigorous programmes of study, completing her Cert Ed., (FE) BSc (Hons) and Adv. Dip Education simultaneously before moving onto her M.Ed.

From there she took further demanding programmes in Human Nutrition, Pharmacology, Neuroscience, Genetics and Immunology. During this time, she was given many prestigious awards for her academic work. It was noted then that Lynne was not afraid of tackling difficult subjects.

She began her law degree but ill health prevented her from pursuing this. However, in this time, she moved from being a foster parent to adoptive parent.

She has been instrumental in setting up projects in the community for disadvantaged groups.

She is a member of the Guild of Health Writers.

Now retired, she lives with her husband in a historic Georgian riverside town in the West Midlands. She enjoys gardening, watching her husband bowling and researching.

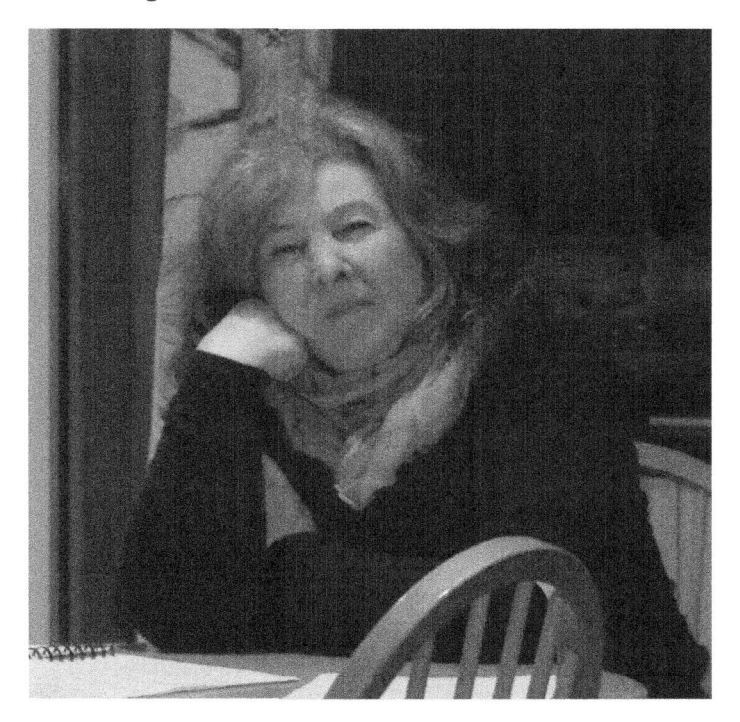

Author Lynne Noble at home

https://quintessentiallylynne.weebly.com/nutritional-medicine.html

Preface

There are just over one billion people worldwide living with elevated or high blood pressure (hypertension) with fewer than one in five having control of this condition.

Controlling high blood pressure is vitally important to achieve. Hypertension is a major cause of morbidity and premature death. It is connected with stroke, heart attack heart failure and cognitive decline.

While some healthy lifestyle changes – such as weight loss, exercise and lower fat diets - may control elevated blood pressure and hypertension, it is not always the case that it does. There are a number of reasons why elevated blood pressure or hypertension occurs and these need to be addressed properly. Some of the medication given to control hypertension is counter-productive.

A case in point is that my husband is happily overweight and is not overly concerned about exercise but has the blood pressure and cholesterol levels of a 20-year-old. His cousin is as thin as a lat and eats like a bird although what he does eat is considered as being the perfect healthy diet. In addition, has an energetic two mile walk every day in order to keep healthy. Surprisingly, he is the one with the high blood pressure.

Symptoms do not always manifest themselves especially in the case of elevated blood pressure. Therefore, the only way to keep track of your blood pressure is to buy a blood pressure monitor known as the sphygmometer.

This is by far the easiest way to keep track of your blood pressure. It is unlikely you will go to the GP for a mainly symptomless condition although anything untoward may be picked up at an appointment for another condition.

There are, of course annual check-ups but these are largely hit and miss affairs. All in all, it is better if you buy your own monitor – known as a sphygmometer – and take more responsibility for your own health. This will avoid the 'white coat hypertension' when an individual's blood pressure rises at the sight of a health professional.

Hypertension may cause some symptoms but these can be vague and are often ignored when life is busy. However, there are some symptoms indicative of high blood pressure which include nosebleeds, severe headaches, arrhythmia (irregular heartbeat), confusion, tiredness, difficulty breathing, blood in the urine, chest pain and blood shot eyes. Some of the symptoms have the potential to be quite severe if the patient is also on blood thinners.

The treatment for blood pressure depends on the stage the blood pressure has reached and into which category. For simplicity's sake GP's normally categorise blood pressure into four stages:

Normal

Mild (pre-hypertension)

Moderate (stage 1)

Severe (stage 2)

Once you have an idea of what category you are in it can be a pleasing challenge to work towards moving to a lower category. Motivation is key in making changes but you need to know your baseline so that you can see how much you have achieved in any allotted time.

It cannot be said enough that the increase in blood pressure that appears to occur alongside the ageing process is not inevitable. Many diseases of older age occur because our nutritional requirements change as we age and we need to adapt our diet to this.

Adaptations to our diet occur throughout our lives although we pay scant attention to this and how it may affect our health. Babies are weaned off milk and onto more solid food. Children are introduced to even greater food choices with encouragement to eat five a day and plenty of protein for growing bodies. Teenage girls especially need to be mindful of the amount of iron in their diet. As the teens are the time of experimentation and plant based diets, reminders may need to be delivered frequently that such diets do not contribute much in the way of iron.

As the ageing process continues, we find that we need less carbohydrate as our tendency to put on weight 'just at the sight of a chocolate muffin' becomes all too obvious.

We have mantras such as 'a moment on the lips, a lifetime on the hips.'

We find we may become arthritic, suffer joint pain, fatigue, sagging skin and lack lustre hair. Do people ever ask themselves why this happens? What mechanisms might be in play here or do they just assume it is an inevitable part of the ageing process and that nothing can be done about it?

It is clearly obvious that if we feed a baby on an adult diet and vice versa that the individual will become ill. This thought takes us nicely into the realisation that lifestyle and not the ageing process, per se, underpins disease of the elderly.

This book has been written to help patients with high blood pressure understand their condition better. You will learn that there is not just one cause; there are numerous causes that underpin this condition. Lifestyle changes which rely heavily on nutrition and its impact on blood pressure will be discussed in detail.

It may surprise you that commonly prescribed medications for high blood pressure are frequently responsible for maintaining high blood pressure. This sounds a strange concept but many medications appear to hold the patient in a chronic state of ill health.

When addressing elevated blood pressure there are a number of medications that can be used. The benefits may be looked at in isolation without considering some of the side effects which may cause the very condition that we are taking the medication to treat.

I see this a lot. Some patients develop anaphylaxis type symptoms to the antihistamines prescribed to treat the condition, for example. Therefore, measures put into place to reduce elevated blood pressure may not necessarily work.

In addition, some medications commonly used to lower blood pressure have the potential to increase visceral fat which would further increase the risk for high blood pressure.

Visceral fat pumps out inflammatory chemicals which can damage the delicate linings of arteries. There are sustained low end levels of inflammation. Arteries become roughened promoting plaque. Blood clots may be triggered in this cascade of events and we need to avoid these at all costs because blood clots are the main cause of stroke and heart attack.

This book is intended to inform you about some of the many causes of high blood pressure and how to address them through bespoke nutrition. I have not ever tried to make adaptations to diet difficult. They have to be something that can be slotted into everyday life without too much thought.

I will try and address each potential cause separately but there is a great deal of overlap between different causes and you may find that a discussion on insufficient electrolytes may encroach into another cause – that of obesity, for example.

Interspersed throughout, there are references to other lifestyle changes which you can make alongside the changes to diet.

Individual lifestyles vary remarkably and not everyone can fit all desirable lifestyle changes into their lives. Others lack motivation and need support or encouragement from others. There is nothing to stop them – or you - from joining a walking group or forming a small group where people create - or adapt - recipes which help to address various aspects of high blood pressure.

As always, I will encourage you to keep a pen and paper to hand so that you can jot relevant information down as you read it.

Causes and risk factors associated with raised blood pressure

As we have already seen there are 4 stages associated with blood pressure. It is helpful to know what these are because, in the fight against hypertension, the responsibility for our health should be a joint one between the health care provider and the individual.

The different stages are better understood when they are tabulated as below.

Description of blood pressure stage	Range
Low blood pressure	Less than 90/60
normal	120/80
Mild (pre-hypertension)	120-139 to 80-89
Moderate (stage 1)	140/90
Severe (stage 2)	Over 140/99

There are a number of risk factors associated with raised blood pressure. These can be grouped into two categories. These can be lifestyle factors and non-lifestyle factors.

While it is easier to see that contributing lifestyle factors can be moderated, it is not so easy to understand that genetic inheritance can also be modified.

Most people believe that genetic influence cannot be changed; that it is set in stone. While the genome – or underlying propensity to a condition – is more or less permanent – the epigenome which produces proteins and other molecules, regulates the genes by turning them on or off on the strands of DNA. The epigenome is influenced heavily by environmental factors - one of the greatest of these is that of nutrition.

Thus, changing your diet can act as a major influencer in turning genes off that are contributing to raised blood pressure.

It is probably useful at this moment to look at some of the risk factors that contribute to high blood pressure. I will try to categorise them into one of the above groups - genetic or environmental influence - but there really is a lot of overlap in ways that gene and the environment interact. They are co-dependent and we have moved far from the concept that if something is written in our DNA then there's nothing that can be done.

Within inherited conditions there can be vast differences in the way a condition is experienced by each member of that family. In some families, medical conditions appear to skip a generation but reappear in the following one. Clearly, if grandparent and grandchild have the same condition and the parent doesn't then we can make a good guess that there are environmental influences at play that protect the parent from displaying symptoms even though they are carrying a gene for a specific condition.

Amenable to life style choice	Probably genetic in origin or unchangeable circumstances
Obesity (but thin people can also suffer from high blood pressure due to inflammatory processes going on. Visceral fat can be found in thin people and makes them vulnerable to inflammatory processes. People who carry a lot of their weight around their hips may be obese but this fat deposition is not associated with inflammation. Some high blood pressure medications do encourage the laying down of visceral fat particularly the diuretics like Furosemide and other non - potassium	Over the age of 65 years The tendency to either a pear or apple shaped form appears to be largely inherited but take note that non-potassium sparing water tablets and steroids enable the deposition of fat around the abdomen.

sparing water tablets	
Food Choices **High salt intake** and **low electrolytes and mineral intake** (primarily magnesium and potassium) **lack of taurine** – an amino acid – may contribute to fluid retention. Taurine helps keep potassium and magnesium in the cells and sodium chloride out of the cells, thus providing its diuretic effect. Taurine is found mainly in shellfish and chicken.	Black African or Black Caribbean descent – appears to be an association with low potassium and diabetes type 2 Some people appear to be salt sensitive and remove salt slowly from their system
Lack of exercise The sort of exercise that is beneficial for those with hypertension is walking where at least part of the walk involves getting slighted out of breath as you do so. Thus walking up a fairly	**Problems which may cause difficulties with exercising** Sometimes there are difficulties with getting adequate exercise. Conditions like arthritis or some form of connective or pulmonary condition

shallow incline or walking at a faster pace than normal would fulfil this criteria. Walking also helps to alleviate stress by using up adrenaline. Adrenaline constricts blood vessels which pushes up blood pressure, Swimming is a very good alternative to walking.	may limit this. It is always worth taking a look at these conditions again especially from a different angle than traditional medicine. Prescribing is limited in many respects and often depends on funding in a particular area or commissioning group. Nutritional medicine has been known to completely cure chronic conditions such as arthritis, for example.
Too many caffeine based drinks Caffeine constricts blood vessels which, in turn, increases blood pressure, There are taurine-based drinks on the market (which help lower blood pressure) or decaffeinated drinks. 'Green drinks' or beetroot juice promote nitric oxide which widens	**Chronic stress or deprivation** – sometimes the job you are doing, the area you live, poor family relationships may contribute to stress and consequently high blood pressure. While not generally insurmountable, these are not aspects of life that have a quick fix to them.

arteries and lowers blood pressure	Looking at options with a trusted professional may be a first step in looking at how to change stressful situations.
Lack of good quality sleep There are many reasons why we do not get good quality sleep such as poor nutrition, lack of exercise, stress and being surrounded by noise and light.	There may be a **hereditary aspect to poor quality sleep** or insomnia of some form. Nevertheless, environmental factors carry most sway. To look at factors most likely to negatively impact sleep, this book may help. Sleep, Perchance to Dream by Lynne D M Noble
Smoking or excess alcohol Nicotine binds to nicotinic acetylcholine receptors in the brain. It speeds up the messages travelling between body and brain. It increases the activity of a number of neurotransmitters. In addition, smoking accelerates	**A familial pattern of high blood pressure** High blood pressure can run in families but even though there may be a vulnerability to it, it is not always clear whether there are some shared environmental factors such as similar dietary intake which could cause this.

arteriosclerosis, (hardening of the arteries) and the formation of plaque in the arteries (atherosclerosis).
Alcohol is initially a stimulant and would keep you awake and elevate your heart rate and blood pressure.

Arteriosclerosis and atherosclerosis due to an **incompetent diet**
Some nutrients like vitamins B3, B6 and B9 are required to complete a certain set of processes in the body in a cycle. In the case of the above mentioned B vitamins they enter a process known as the Methionine Cycle. Without adequate nutrition, this cycle cannot be completed and plaque will build up in the arteries.
Antioxidants are required

to attenuate inflammation which is damaging to delicate inner linings of arteries.	

Medications - there are many medications which directly or indirectly can cause high blood pressure. These include:
    Non potassium sparing diuretics
    Steroids
    Antihistamines
    Many medications prescribed for high blood pressure.	

The table provides a simple overview and issues raised will be covered in more detail later in this book.

I have always found that individuals with high blood pressure are less likely to make the necessary changes if they do not understand the underlying reasons for these.

How, for example, does obesity contribute to elevated blood pressure? From there, we can understand the anxious patient who has tried for years to lose weight and has not managed to achieve this at all.

Now that we have had a simple overview of the main causes of hypertension, it would be judicious to look at each category in more detail. I will look at the subject of obesity first. It is one of the main factors that health professionals consider in looking for a cause for hypertension. Losing weight can help lower blood pressure but in some people it does not work. Calorie restrictive diets has the potential to make hypertension worse.

Obesity

Calorie restrictive diets do not work. They leave people hungry, deprived of essential nutrients and often suffering the effects of sub-nutrition. Many people who have been on calorie restricting diets have sagging skin. This is because they are limiting the essential nutrients to maintain connective tissue and underlying musculature.

One interesting study has found that a deficiency of electrolytes like potassium is linked to obesity. When people restrict their calories one of the nutrients that tends to be restricted is potassium.

The role of potassium in lowering blood pressure and reducing obesity deserves a great deal of attention. It is to this subject we will now turn.

Potassium, the overlooked mineral in the war against obesity and blood pressure

While most studies focus on calorie reduction of carbohydrates and fat to reduce the impact of metabolic syndrome – which includes abdominal obesity and elevated blood pressure - more recent studies[1] have looked at the impact of electrolytes in this process. In particular, increments in dietary potassium has been found to predict weight loss during treatment of metabolic syndrome and obesity.

Potassium has not generally been seen as a major contributor in responding to metabolic syndrome. Most people have heard of potassium but there has been little in the media to suggest that there is a deficiency of this mineral cum electrolyte in the population as a whole.

However, potassium is essential for enabling your muscles to work effectively. This includes muscles like your heart and the ones that control breathing.

Individuals with low potassium levels often have digestive problems like slow bowel transit which may result in constipation and impaction. Sedate walking

---

[1] https://www.ncbi.nlm.nih.gov/pmc/articles/PMC6627830/#:~:text=It%20is%20notable%20that%20the,and%20in%20overall%20caloric%20intake.

may be problematical; legs may feel heavy and taking steps an effort.

Brain fog and the inability to remember recent events may also be due to low potassium levels. You may not feel motivated to do much exercise either – hardly helpful in the battle against hypertension.

Potassium, along with magnesium, balances the fluid in your body so a diet which is sufficient in both these minerals should address oedema which is caused by a deficiency of them. My expectation is that deficiencies of either potassium or magnesium will be one of the more likely causes of elevated blood pressure. Excess fluid will, of course, elevate blood pressure as the heart has more fluid to pump around the body.

Excessive fluid in the tissues has a tendency to make them quite tender when touched and may be one of the symptoms that will alert you to an imbalance of electrolytes in the system.

Initially then, the fluid loss caused by diuretics will lower blood pressure as there is less fluid for the heart to pump. However, this is only a temporary measure. The half-life of diuretics is approximately 6 hours at which point you may feel dehydrated or thirsty and drink more to relieve this feeling. Indeed, it would not be wise to keep yourself in a state of dehydration. It is simply not healthy.

In addition, as the diuretics will have relieved you (no pun intended) of valuable electrolytes and minerals you will probably be craving foods that contain these nutrients that you have now become deficient in.

The nutrients that diuretics can cause a deficiency of are:

    Potassium

    Magnesium

    Zinc

Taking diuretics really does make it very difficult to lose weight.

The fat deposition around the visceral organs caused by low potassium also pumps out inflammatory chemicals. Inflammation is always accompanied by leaky vessels and oedema.

Obese individuals also fall victim to the Renin-Angiotensin System (RAS) which is an important hormone mechanism that contributes to hypertension in obese individuals.

The RAS helps regulate:

    Blood pressure

    Fluid

    Electrolyte balance

    Systemic vascular resistance

When activated it increases:

    Sodium reabsorption

    Water reabsorption

    Vascular tone

All of which contributes to high blood pressure.

The RAS is activated by sudden drops in blood pressure such as those you would find when fluid is lost through the use of diuretics.

Thus as soon as fluid is lost through the use of diuretics the RAS kicks in to make sure that sodium and water is reabsorbed again thus negating the effects of diuretics.

It is an efficient feedback loop to the insult of diuretics although the nutrients lost through the use of diuretics are not always replaced. It is not unusual to find that patients on diuretic therapy are deficient in potassium.

To prevent the RAS from doing its job, beta blockers were invented. They were the original RAS system inhibitors. They blocked adrenaline and had some interesting side effects like turning your finger nails black. Other symptoms include:

    Poor circulation with cold fingers and toes

Slow heartbeat

Gastrointestinal symptoms such as bloating, constipation or diarrhoea

Muscle weakness

Insomnia

Weight gain

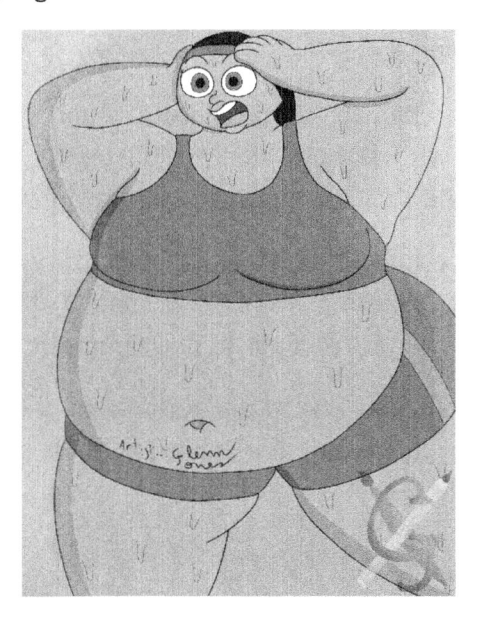

Weight gain is a side effect of beta blockers

This is not a definitive list.

However, beta blockers exert their effects by:

>Lowering metabolic rate so that you don't burn as many calories

>Increasing appetite

>Causing fat to accumulate around your belly (found with all beta blockers but more so with the older one such as Atenolol and Metroprol).

The negative impact of diuretics on obesity and health are so far reaching that it is useful to see the interconnectedness of it all in diagrammatic form.

Most beta blockers end in the suffix 'olol' and are easily identified in this way. The most common one used is Propranolol.

Diagram to show the impact of thiazide diuretics on obesity and hypertension

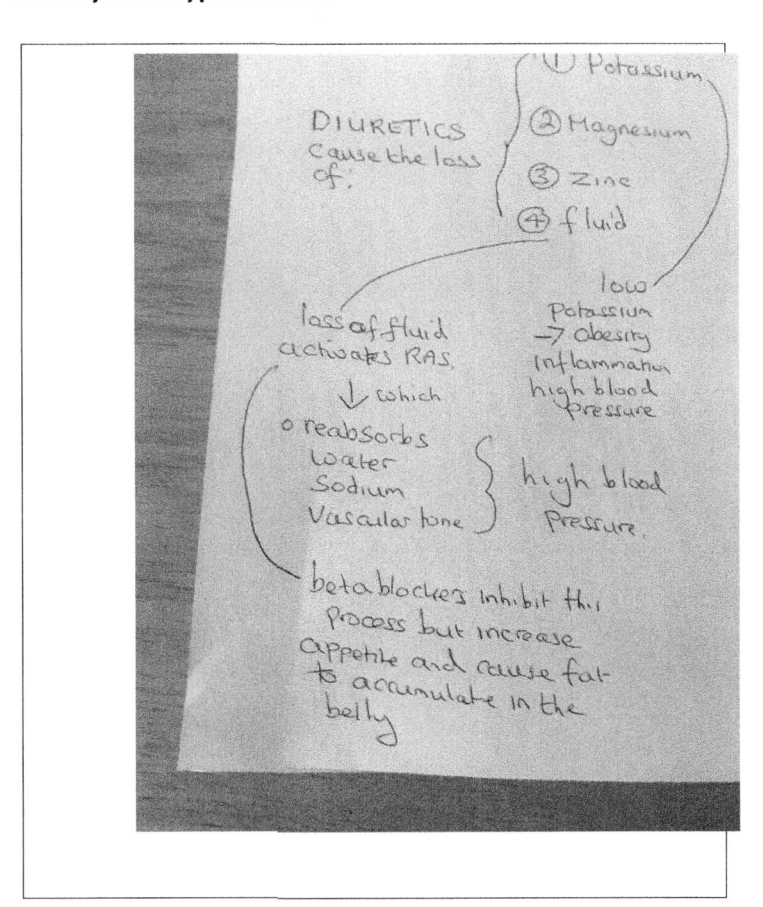

DIURETICS Cause the loss of:
1. Potassium
2. Magnesium
3. Zinc
4. fluid

low Potassium → obesity
Inflammation
high blood pressure

loss of fluid activates RAS,
↓ which
○ reabsorbs water
  Sodium
  Vascular tone
} high blood pressure.

beta blockers inhibit this process but increase appetite and cause fat to accumulate in the belly

It would be useful to go one step further and look at the impact of low potassium, low magnesium levels (hypomagnesia) and low zinc levels.

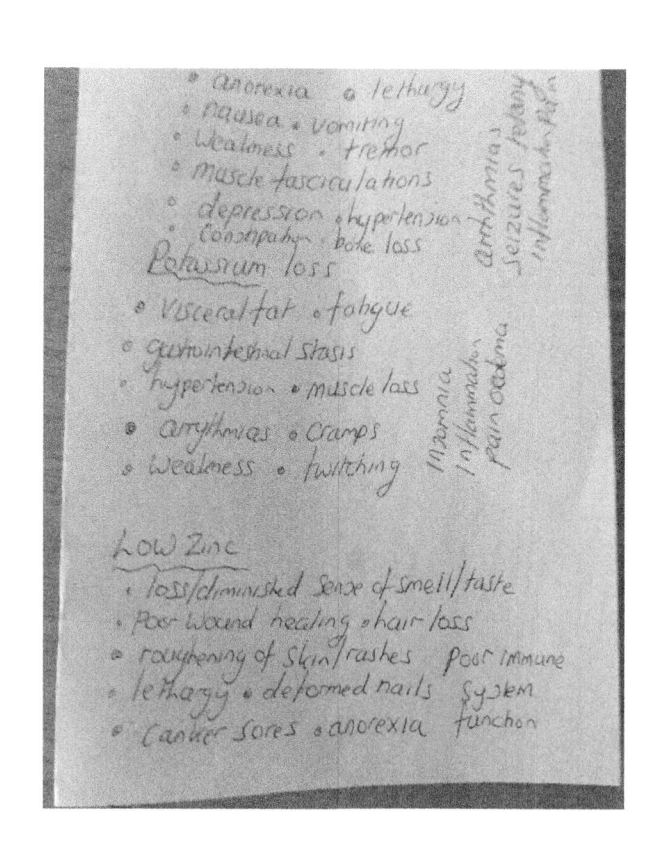

- anorexia
- nausea
- weakness
- muscle fasciculations
- depression
- constipation
- lethargy
- vomiting
- tremor
- hypertension
- bone loss
- arrhythmias
- seizures
- tetany
- inflammation pain

Potassium loss

- visceral fat
- gastrointestinal stasis
- hypertension
- arrhythmias
- weakness
- fatigue
- muscle loss
- cramps
- twitching
- insomnia
- inflammation
- pain oedema

Low Zinc

- loss/diminished sense of smell/taste
- poor wound healing
- hair loss
- roughening of skin/rashes
- lethargy
- deformed nails
- canker sores
- anorexia
- poor immune system function

Studies have shown that vast swathes of the population are deficient in magnesium and potassium. Recently the dietary recommended intake for potassium was increased from 2700mg to 4700mg daily.

It was thought that this was easily achievable and that potassium intake was not a problem.

However, I would take issue with that. It is not that easy to ingest 4700 of potassium daily – it might be worth totting up how much you do have for about three days. In addition, if are prescribed diuretics then most of that potassium will be flushed away.

Indeed, other studies[2] have shown that only 10% of men reach their RDI of potassium and for women that figure drops to 1%.

Further, potassium cannot be used if there is not sufficient magnesium available and most people do not have enough dietary magnesium as it is.

The recommended daily amount of magnesium is 300mg daily but magnesium is flushed – along with

---

[2] https://pubmed.ncbi.nlm.nih.gov/22322920/

potassium and zinc – out of the body with the use of diuretics. There are many studies that suggest that daily intake of magnesium should equal that of the Recommended Daily Intake (RDI) of calcium. This currently stands at 800mg.

Although there are a number of symptoms associated with each deficiency, you don't have to have all the symptoms to qualify for a deficiency. Genetic variation means that different people will manifest a unique cluster of varied symptoms.

The outcome of taking diuretics may be a temporary loss of weight and blood pressure but as low potassium continues, it will contribute to abdominal obesity – or what is quaintly known as a protuberant abdomen - inflammation, elevated blood pressure and muscle breakdown.

In African Americans, low potassium levels were particularly associated with an increased incidence of diabetes type 2.[3]

So how easy is it to get sufficient potassium and magnesium in your diet? Well, it is not that easy if you are elderly, have a poor appetite (appetites diminish as we age), not a particular lover of fresh fruit or veg or

---

[3] https://pubmed.ncbi.nlm.nih.gov/22322920/

take certain medications like diuretics which are non-potassium sparing.

To round up a collection of symptoms related to potassium deficiency makes it easier to identify.

- Protuberant abdomen
- Generalised weakness
- Impaired insulin production resulting in high blood sugar levels
- Muscle cramps and spasms
- Bloating and gastrointestinal discomfort due to poor gut motility
- Palpitation
- Muscle aches and stiffness
- Tingling and numbness

Dr Houston argues that hypertension is a 'correct and chronic dysregulated vascular response to infinite insults to the blood vessel. He cities:

- Inflammation
- Oxidative stress
- Vascular immune dysfunction

as the culprits.

Now Dr Houston[4] states that elevated blood pressure is one among multiple responses to endothelial dysfunction and vascular smooth muscle dysfunction both of which precede the development of hypertension by decades.

Sadly, the use of diuretics aids this process. Potassium and magnesium are needed in adequate amounts to reduce inflammation. Zinc is an effective antioxidant.

For a short term gain in lowering blood pressure through the use of diuretics, there is chronic ill health brewing as the subtler impact of these nutrient deficiencies begin to exert their effect.

I should also add to Dr Houston's list of insults to blood vessels. We cannot forget salt can cause inflammation.

Of course a little in the diet is fine but we were never meant to sprinkle our food liberally with the stuff or eat huge amounts of processed foods which have salt added to them.

Sufficient potassium aids the removal of salt from inside the cells where it would cause them to swell, causing

---

[4] **ttps://www.ncbi.nlm.nih.gov/pmc/articles/PMC3989080/**

pain. Indeed, I believe that much of the pain that we feel nowadays is from the impact of too much salt and too little potassium and magnesium in the diet to create a healthy balance of electrolytes.

It is useful at this point to identify foods which are rich in potassium, magnesium and zinc since these are lost through the use of diuretics. I will also add a table of natural beta blockers.

Table of potassium containing foods

RDA adults = 3600 – 4700 mg

Food source   **amount (mg) per portion**

avocado	485mg of potassium per 100g
potatoes	421/100g
Kidney beans/lentils cooked	405/100g
mushrooms	318/100g
Cooked spinach	270/100g
peas	244/100g
Tomato juice	229/100ml
milk	150/100g

Potassium is found in many foods especially fruit and vegetables and it is argued that everyone would be taking in enough. However, this is not the case and potassium deficiency is rife. More so if you are taking diuretics or on a weight reducing diet which is a calorie restricted one.

Table of Magnesium containing foods

RDA adults =   350 - 800mg

Food source   amount (mg) per portion

Food source	Amount
Peanuts(and most nuts)	63mg/100g
spinach	78mg/100g
70% dark chocolate	50mg//25g
3.5 oz baked potato	43mg
yogurt	12mg/100g
2 slices of whole wheat bread	46mg
2 shredded wheat	46mg
almonds	80mg/25g

Potassium requires sufficient magnesium to be able to undertake its functions in the body. Nuts – especially almonds – are an excellent source of magnesium

Table of popular Zinc containing foods

(RDA adults = 8-11mg daily)

Food source   **mg per serving**

oysters	74mg/3 oz serving
Braised beef	7mg/3 oz
Baked beans	2.9mg/100g
Beef patty	5.3mg/3 oz serving
dark meat chicken	2.4/3 oz serving
milk	1mg/200ml
Yogurt	1.7/200ml
Kidney beans	0.9mg/150g

Zinc is not found in any great amount in foods of plant origin. Zinc binds to phytates in plant sources and renders it unabsorbable. People on plant based diets - like vegans or vegetarians - are at particular risk of zinc deficiency.

Only enough zinc is stored in the body to last one day and if you are taking diuretics this will be lost along with any allegedly excess fluid.

Although zinc is normally associated as being required for optimum immune system function, it has also been found that lower than normal zinc levels may contribute to hypertension. It does this by altering the way the kidneys hand sodium.

Indirectly, by keep infection away, the risk of inflammatory processes – which can activate the RAS – are also kept low.

Natural beta blockers – which prevent activation of the RAS system – do exist and are listed below.

Natural Beta Blockers

Magnesium

Omega 3

Co-enzyme Q 10

Berberine

Green leafy vegetables

Nuts and seeds

Meat and poultry

These are good substitutes for those 'olol' medications indicative of beta blockers.

There aren't that many sources of omega 3. The two main animal sources are known as EPA and DHA for short. They have powerful anti-inflammatory effect in the body.

Oily fish such as mackerel, sardine and salmon are generally the best food sources of this poly unsaturated fatty acid.

Some foods are fortified with omega e such as eggs where hens are fed on a high omega 3 diet.

Vegetables are a good source of ala-linolenic acid known as ALA. Green leafy vegetables are a good source. While its anti-inflammatory effects are not as great as EPA and DHA, it is still vitally important to eat plenty of green leafy vegetables. I include at least one generous portion daily.

Other sources of ALA are nuts and seeds and this would include chia and flax seeds. Consequently, nut oils, although expensive, are also a good source.

Oils are delicate and go rancid easily. This occurs because of a chemical reaction that causes the fat molecules in the oil to degenerate. Exposure, to heat, air and light will hasten this process so oils need to be stored in the cool, with the lid tightly on and in the refrigerator.

Sesame and walnut oil appear be particularly susceptible to going rancid. Buy small bottles that can be used quickly. Tip some over soup, dip your bread in it, feed it to your chickens if you have a little that you are not needing to use for a while.

Co-enzyme Q10 – which I shall just refer to as Q10 from now on – is a substance that your body makes in tiny organelles present in every cell. It helps generate energy and so they are known as the power houses of each cell.

In addition, Q10 protects from bacterial and viral infections and oxidative stress.

Unfortunately, as you age, Q10 production begins to decline.

Many conditions associated with older age appear to be connected to a deficiency of Q10 and these conditions include:

    Diabetes

    Degenerative brain disorders

    Some cancers

Heart disease

There are a number of reasons why the production of Q10 declines apart from the ageing process. These include:

Inadequate vitamin B6 since the nucleus of Q10 - which contains tyrosine - is dependent on the availability vitamin B6 for its synthesis.

Oxidative stress occurs when there is an imbalance of the production of oxygen reactive species (ROS) in cells and tissues and the body's ability to neutralise them

Genetic defects which prevent the making or using of Q10

Statin treatment – statins prevent the synthesis of Q10.

Increased demand due to disease

Although it is fairly simple to take a vitamin B complex supplement, in order to allow for the synthesis of Q10's nucleus, it is always useful to have an idea of which foods contain which nutrients.

Vitamin B6 is found in

    Peanuts

Fish

Wheat germ

Oats

Soya beans

Some fortified breakfast cereal

Bananas

milk

It would be difficult not to get enough vitamin B6 unless you were a very picky eater.

Now, vitamin B6 is a water soluble vitamin and vulnerable to being flushed out of the body too. However, studies have shown that although chronic diuretic use is associated with a significant increase in a protein called homocysteine, vitamin B6 levels do not appear to be affected.

Homocysteine can have a devastating impact on the body. It is associated with heart disease and stroke. It is part of a cycle in the body and thus required. However, it presents only briefly provided there are adequate amounts of vitamin B6, folate and vitamin B12.

Studies show that whilst there is no significant change in vitamin B6 and B12 concentrations, there is a significant decrease in red blood cell folate concentration.

Folate is found in a wide variety of foods so the impact of diuretics on blood cell folate concentration is to be taken very seriously.

In addition, to help prevent homocysteine build up, a folate deficiency can also cause:

    muscle weakness

    pins and needles, tingling, burning, peripheral neuropathy, numbness

    tiredness, lethargy or fatigue

Table showing foods containing folate[5]

Food	Micrograms (mcg) DFE per serving	Percent DV*
Beef liver, braised, 3 ounces	215	54
Spinach, boiled, ½ cup	131	33
Black-eyed peas (cowpeas), boiled, ½ cup	105	26
Breakfast cereals, fortified with 25% of the DV†	100	25
Rice, white, medium-grain, cooked, ½ cup†	90	22
Asparagus, boiled, 4 spears	89	22
Brussels sprouts, frozen, boiled, ½ cup	78	20
Spaghetti, cooked, enriched, ½ cup†	74	19
Lettuce, romaine, shredded, 1 cup	64	16
Avocado, raw, sliced, ½ cup	59	15
Spinach, raw, 1 cup	58	15
Broccoli, chopped, frozen, cooked, ½ cup	52	13
Mustard greens, chopped, frozen, boiled, ½ cup	52	13
Bread, white, 1 slice†	50	13
Green peas, frozen, boiled, ½ cup	47	12
Kidney beans, canned, ½ cup	46	12
Wheat germ, 2 tablespoons	40	10
Tomato juice, canned, ¾ cup	36	9
Crab, Dungeness, 3 ounces	36	9
Orange juice, ¾ cup	35	9
Turnip greens, frozen, boiled, ½ cup	32	8

---

[5] https://ods.od.nih.gov/factsheets/Folate-HealthProfessional/#:~:text=Folate%20is%20naturally%20present%20in,)%20%5B4%2C12%5D.

Inflammatory markers

Hypertension is associated with an inflammatory marker known as C-reactive protein. When you go to the GP then one of the blood tests that may be ordered is for C-reactive protein.

Raised C- reactive protein -= inflammation

It has been found that systemic low grade inflammation precedes hypertension.

Inflammation is known to stimulate the Renin Angiotensin Aldosterone System along with salt and oxidative stress. This would lead to the retention of salt and fluid.

Inflammation can also alter the rates and synthesis of substances which regulate blood vessel diameter.

One of these substances is Nitric Oxide. Most people have heard of nitric oxide in connection with the medication given to those who have angina.

Nitric oxide, in the body, is produced to help blood vessels dilate which causes a drop in blood pressure. Inflammation appears to dysregulate the synthesis of nitric oxide causing blood pressure to rise in the process.

Fortunately, for us there are foods which promote nitric oxide levels. These include beetroot, nuts, leafy green vegetables, dark chocolate, garlic and meat.

Stimulants of the RAAS

salt	Oxidative stress	Inflammation found in tissue repair	Inflammation found in infection

⬇

Stimulates the RAAS

Why does infection cause inflammation?

During infection certain immune cells from your innate system (the defence system you were born with) will arrive at the site of infection and pour toxic chemicals on the pathogen in order to eliminate it.

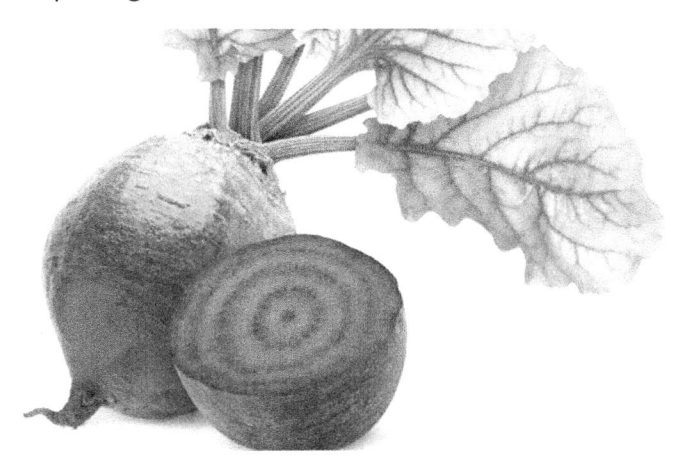

Beetroot is a great vegetable for dilating blood vessels, thus lowering blood pressure.

The immune system has a tendency to go overboard and swamp the infected area with immune cells. One of the main substances that is released is hydrogen peroxide (yes, that stuff used to bleach hair),

When neutrophils – one of the body's first responders - detect hydrogen peroxide they rush to the site of injury or infection. They will attack foreign invaders, remove any damaged tissue and initiate an inflammatory process designed to bring other healing substances to the site of injury.

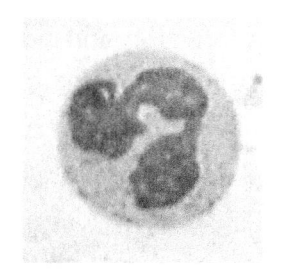

A neutrophil is attracted to the site of injury when it detects hydrogen peroxide.

Neutrophils produce their own hydrogen peroxide but it is also produced during day to day metabolic processes. Thus when neutrophils have been attracted to a site of injury or inflammation, they release hydrogen peroxide signalling other neutrophils to join them.

Neutrophils have an arsenal of weapons at their disposal including Reactive Oxygen Species (ROS). Sometimes they are called oxygen radicals or free radicals.

A build-up of these will cause damage to DNA, RNA and proteins. They may even cause the demise of the cell. In order to keep levels down then plentiful antioxidants are required in the diet.

To this end we are often to eat 5 a day. We are informed that different coloured fruit and vegetables will keep us healthy.

For someone who likes fruit and copious amounts of vegetables (cooked for the minimum time possible) this does not present a problem. However, not everyone does yet no-one is ever told that there are some great antioxidants that are found in animal products which can be more effective than the antioxidants found in fruit and vegetables.

Further, a diet high in plant foods contains phytic acid. Phytic acid enables phosphorus to be stored in a number of plants including seeds, nuts and beans.

However, too much phytic acid is detrimental to health. It binds to other minerals including:

zinc

manganese

calcium

magnesium

iron

chromium

When phytic acid binds to minerals it forms phytates and these cannot be broken down so that we can use these minerals they are bound to. We simply do not have the enzymes to do so.

For this reason, phytic acid is referred to as an anti – nutrient and it is generally found in raw and unprocessed plant based diets.

Thus what initially appears to be a very healthy diet may cause problems in some people.

To reduce the impact of phytic acid then:

    fermenting

    sprouting

    baking

    processing

    soaking

    cooking

all help to reduce the binding of minerals which are required to reduce blood pressure or blood sugar levels.

Garlic and onions also enhance the absorption of minerals.

While cooking may destroy some vitamin C, it does not destroy the mineral content of food although some may leach out into the cooking water.

Whole grains not only contain phytic acid but substances called saponins and lectins.

Saponins and lectins are also referred to as anti-nutrients and they too, can have a detrimental impact on blood pressure and health in general.

Lectins

Lectins are associated with auto-immune disease, inflammation and obesity. They are proteins that attach themselves to carbohydrates and then cells.

DLJ Freed (1999) stated that many lectins are 'toxic, inflammatory or both.' He maintains that they cause endothelial dysfunction but that removal of lectins can restore the endothelium and reverse high blood pressure, diabetes and obesity.

Some people do appear to be particularly susceptible to lectins. They are not easily digested and can sit heavily on the stomach to those susceptible to their effects. When they bind to cells lining the digestive tract they prevent the growth of intestinal flora which is required for gut motility.

It is not therefore true that a high fibre diet is good for constipation in all people.

On a more positive side, lectins are able to cause cancer cell death.

If you do like the taste of high lectin foods but suffer from their side effects, then cooking at high heat does inactivate them.

Saponins

These are also classed as anti-nutrients if they are the bitter form (known as steroid or triterpene glycosides). These compounds help to protect the plant from being eaten by insects as well as offer some protection against bacteria. However, in humans they inhibit enzymes which are required for metabolic and digestive processes.

Robb Wolf, author of The Paleo Solution says that saponins punch holes in the membranes of microvilli cells This is irritating to the immune system. Indeed, saponins are used in vaccine research as they help the body to mount a much more powerful immune response.

You can easily recognise when plants contain saponins. When you cook them they release foam and needs to be skimmed off as the food is being cooked.

Saponins are not always anti-nutrients and as long as they do not belong to the bitter class of saponins, help reduce blood pressure quite considerably in some people. (we have always got to consider genetic variability). They have been found to do this by blocking circulating and tissue RAAS.

So, plant diets may not be the best move for some people who are susceptible to plant based substances although they will work well for some people. We will look at non plant based sources of antioxidants shortly.

Saponins may be useful for some people to try with the aim of lowering blood pressure and for others they can be problematical.

This is what we would expect because everyone is different and only trial and error will determine whether eating foods will help lower your blood pressure. However, if you are one of the lucky ones who respond to foods containing saponins they can dramatically reduce blood pressure by blocking tissue and systemic RAA's.

These foods contain saponins:

- legumes, lentils and peas
- asparagus
- spinach
- onion
- garlic
- tea
- oats
- ginseng
- liquorice
- soy beans

It may help to look at RAAS again and build upon the information already learned about this system.

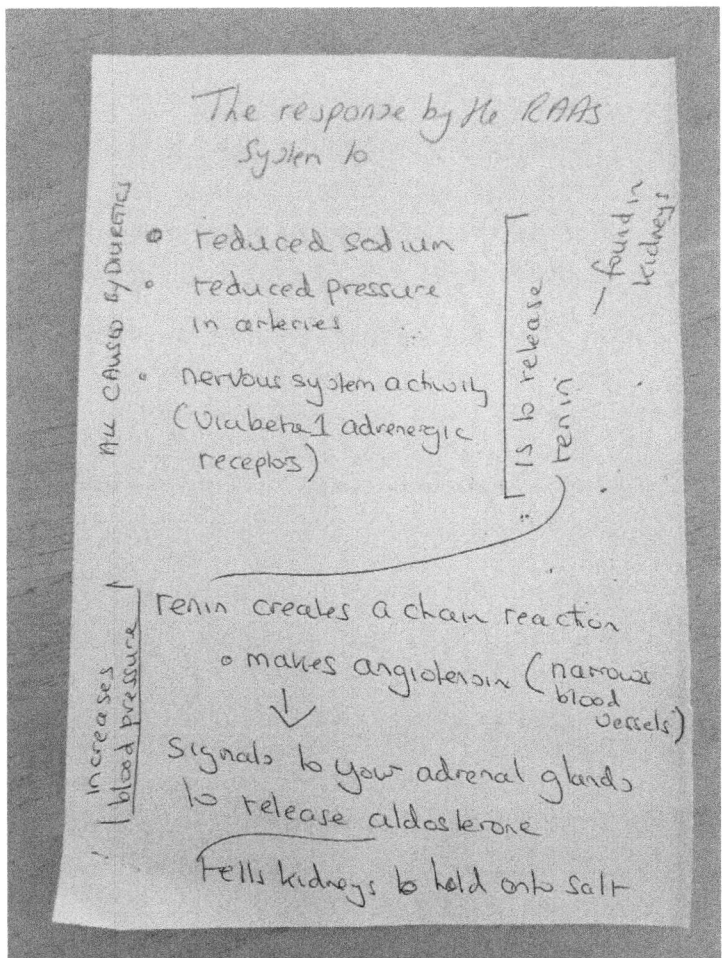

> **The response by the RAAS System to**
>
> *All caused by Diuretics* {
> - reduced sodium
> - reduced pressure in arteries
> - nervous system activity (via beta 1 adrenergic receptors)
> } *is to release renin* — found in kidneys
>
> *Increases blood pressure* {
> Renin creates a chain reaction
> - makes angiotensin (narrows blood vessels)
>   ↓
> Signals to your adrenal glands to release aldosterone
> Tells kidneys to hold onto salt

When the RAAS system detects changes in blood pressure, it releases renin found in the kidneys.

Renin helps control blood pressure and if it drops too low then it sets off a set of chain reactions.

Firstly, it makes a substance called angiotensin which narrows blood vessels. This raises blood pressure.

This signals your adrenal gland to release aldosterone which tells kidneys to hold onto salt. Salt holds onto fluid so the heart has to pump more fluid around the body which, of course increases blood pressure.

In fact, the feedback loop is very effective and will overcome any attempt by diuretics to lower your blood pressure, within hours.

The therapeutic effect of Furosemide (Lasix) is 6-8 hours.

Indapomide, another popular diuretic for the treatment of high blood pressure has a therapeutic effect of 16 hours.

Clearly it is not good to prescribe diuretics which remove vital electrolytes from someone's system and then not be concerned that for some part of the day, the RAAS will have placed the patient back into a state of high blood pressure.

Non plant sources of antioxidants

Zinc, iron, manganese, selenium and copper are all components of antioxidant enzymes. These antioxidant enzymes are found in:

seafood

offal

lean meat

milk

While it is always preferable to have antioxidants from a wide range of both plant and animal sources, this is not always possible. There are people who eat a high fat, high protein diet not dissimilar to the Atkins Diet and they do very well on it.

The French are renowned for eating diets which do not contain many vegetables and yet the French Paradox - high fat diet accompanied by low blood pressure – is well known.

For hundreds of years we have not eaten diets as high in fruit and vegetables as we are urged to now and it has not been detrimental. The Victorians were known to eat diets heavy in butter, cream eggs and animal fat and were a healthy people. Heart disease nor high blood pressure were rife.

There could be a number of reasons for this. It could be worth exploring another disadvantage of eating fruit and why saturated animal fats are actually good for you.

Firstly, though, we have mentioned that renin and aldosterone do impact blood pressure. When you attend the GP and high blood pressure is identified, blood tests will be taken and these can point to which part of your system is contributing to your high blood pressure.

Table showing how blood tests can point to causes of high blood pressure

High renin, low aldosterone	Sensitive to salt
Low renin, high aldosterone	Adrenal glands aren't working properly
High renin and high aldosterone	Possibly a problem with the kidneys

Fructose, the sugar in fruit, may contribute to high blood pressure

Fructose is not just found in fruit; it is also found in vegetables but fructose content will be higher in fruit.

Fructose actually reduces the production of nitric oxide. Nitric oxide, as we have already seen helps the blood vessels dilate thus lowering blood pressure.

Fructose is also known to raise uric acid in the blood. Uric acid is a waste product. It is a by-product of purines which are formed from the breakdown of fructose. Studies show that minutes after a high fructose corn syrup soda is drunk, uric acid levels rise.

The presence of uric acid is associated with raised blood pressure.

Fructose also instructs the kidneys to hold onto more salt. Salt, of course, attracts water so that the fluid volume rises which ultimately impacts high blood pressure.

So while fruit may be useful in replacing potassium lost if diuretics are used to try and lower blood pressure, it may raise blood pressure by other mechanisms.

If diuretics can be avoided, then this means that the reliance on fruit to replace lost potassium, is not so important.

Fructose –fruit sugar- is taken up by the liver and cannot be used for biosynthesis. As such it is promptly converted to a substrate used for making new fat cells.

If you suffer from metabolic syndrome, then you may have to consider lowering your fruit intake or just choosing fruit which are considered to be low fructose.

Fructose also contributes susceptibility to non-alcoholic fatty liver disease.

High fructose foods include:

    apples

grapes

watermelon

asparagus

zucchini

peas

Lower fructose foods include:

bananas

blueberries

strawberries

carrots

green beans

lettuce

There are also many foods that contain hidden sources of fructose.

You need to start label watching. If the product you wish to buy contains:

molasses

palm or coconut sugar

    fructose

    high fructose corn syrup

    agave syrup

    honey

    invert sugar

    sorghum[6]

    maple syrup or maple-flavoured syrup

then you need to find a substitute.

The flapjack that you buy from the supermarket may contain fructose but the one you make at home is unlikely to. Homemade is often best.

You might be surprised to find out how many common food stuffs contain high fructose corn syrup. It is a slow poison and will in the meantime make you look not one bit attractive.

Anyway, here is a list of the more common foods containing high fructose corn syrup.

    Sweetened yogurt

    Salad dressing

    Some brands of bread

---

[6] Sorghum is a plant with diverse uses including animal fodder and biofuel. It is also grown for its sugar content

- Canned fruit
- Granola bars
- Juice
- Junk foods like pizzas and ready meals
- Snack bars
- Cereal bars
- Nutrition bars

Now please do not think that I am saying do not ever have a granola bar again. I am not saying that at all.

Just find one that does not contain a form of fructose or better still make your own.

Fructose is a major contributor to metabolic syndrome and should be avoided at all costs. It is quite possible to lose weight eating - weight for weight - the same food only one is sweetened with glucose and the other fructose.

It will be helpful to copy this Fructose Malabsorption chart out and keep it with you. It will be a reminder of just how ubiquitous fructose is.

Fructose Malabsorption Sugar Chart

AVOID!!!	OK	Maybe?
Agave Syrup	Cane Sugar	Barley Malt Syrup
Aspartame	Confectioners Sugar	Beet Sugar
Brown Sugar	Dextrin	Brown Rice Syrup
Corn Starch	Dextrose	Date Sugar
Corn Sugar	Evaporated Cane Sugar	Maple Syrup
Corn Syrup	Glucose	Raffinose
Corn Syrup Solids	Raw Sugar	Sucrose
Fructose	Stevia	Xylitol
Fruit Juice Sweeteners	Table Sugar (if not beet sugar)	
High Fructose Corn Syrup		
Honey		
Inverted Sugar		
Isoglucose		
Isomalt		
Levulose		
Malitol		
Molasses		
Molasses Sugar		
Saccharin		
Sorbitol		
Splenda		
Sucralose		
Sucrose Syrups		

As you can see, some diets stated as being healthy are not always, it would depend very much on the medical condition that you are trying to address.

Saturated fats are good for you, most vegetable oils are not

Saturated fats are those wonderful fats that are generally solid at room temperature. This includes:

- lard
- butter
- dripping
- cream

Saturated fats do not create reactive oxygen species and therefore are not inflammatory in nature. This may well explain why the Victorians were such a healthy people.

These fats have lots of important vitamins in them that vegetable oils do not. They are important sources of vitamin A and D which are vital for a healthy immune system.

Vitamin D helps to reduce inflammation and is known to lower blood pressure.

All in all, saturated fats are healthy fats.

In contrast many of the vegetable oils on the market are omega 6 poly unsaturated fatty acids and they do have the potential to cause severe and chronic inflammation.

Unfortunately, they are ubiquitous. They are used generously in the kitchen and added to most processed foods that you can buy today from a 'healthy' flapjack to a tin of soup. Where once chips were cooked in dripping, they are now cooked in sunflower oil.

We are in the midst of a tsunami of chronic conditions including metabolic syndrome and its associated high blood pressure.

How do Omega 6 PUFA's cause inflammatory conditions and raise blood pressure?

Omega 6 PUFA's can be highly inflammatory in nature as they can produce arachidonic acid. Some inflammation is required for healing damaged tissues but often inflammation becomes out of control and it is then that it causes problems. PUFA's and arachidonic acid deserve more attention when looking at food substances which may help to progress lipoedema.

Arichidonic acid is a polyunsaturated omega-6 fatty acid. It is found in the membranes of the body's cells and is particularly abundant in the brain, muscles and liver. It is a key inflammatory intermediate and can act as a vasodilator. This means it can widen blood vessels which would help lower blood pressure but please read on.

Arichidonic acid has many beneficial roles in the body. It will not cause inflammation unless tiny particles, called electrons, try and disrupt the stability of other electrons found in the fat that forms part of the cell membranes. Eating plenty of antioxidants would prevent this from happening but our current diets are wanting in that:

> We are eating more and more of the omega 6 polyunsaturated fatty acids in our diets than ever before

> Our diets lack enough of the foods which have antioxidant capacity

> The imbalance of antioxidants to arachidonic acid if you are taking in excessive omega 6 PUFA's will elevate blood pressure.

The test

Arachidonic acid can be metabolised to both anti-inflammatory and proinflammatory eicanosoids. It is quite likely that if you suffer from joint pain, bronchoconstriction, microvascular permeability, high blood pressure, metabolic syndrome, lymphoedema, certain cancers – and many more - that arachidonic acid has been converted to a pro-inflammatory compound in your body.

> Eicanosoids are a class of compounds (like leukotrienes and prostaglandins) which are synthesised from poly unsaturated fatty acids (PUFA's) - like arachidonic acid – and that are involved in cellular activity. They are lipid mediators of inflammation.

In fact, a study[7] on lymphoedema in breast cancer patients has supported the connection between raised omega 6 PUFA's and lymphoedema which is an inflammatory condition.

The study demonstrated that breast cancer survivors with lymphoedema had elevated PUFA's, arachidonic acid, fatty acid desaturase enzyme activity indices and EPA in serum phospholipids.

The study concluded that the extent of fatty acid composition might be related to the risk of secondary lymphoedema in breast cancer survivors.

Where are PUFA's found?

---

[7] https://www.ncbi.nlm.nih.gov/pubmed/27041742

Sources of PUFA's are Canola oil, grapeseed oil, corn oil, soybean oil, peanut oil among others.

There are plenty of hidden sources – granola, crisps, energy bars, flax seeds and commercially raised poultry, beef and eggs all contain PUFA's.

In fact, our consumption of PUFA's has risen dramatically since their introduction into our diets. They have now replaced the more stable saturated fats such as lard, dripping and butter that were the mainstay of the UK diet until around the early 1970's when the apparently 'healthy' benefits of polyunsaturated fatty acids were heavily marketed and included in many ready meals and snacks.

Adenosine is a natural suppressor of arachidonic acid release and leukotriene biosynthesis. A potent natural source of adenosine is brewer's yeast. However, it competes with protein for absorption so it is better taken before food. As it also makes you feel sleepy – it is an inhibitory neurotransmitter – the perfect time to take it is before bedtime.

Brewers' yeast can be sprinkled over food. It is slightly bitter but a debittered type can be bought. It is also available in tablet form and is generally reasonable in price, however it comes. It is also a source of the vitamin B complex.

Unfortunately, oils which are rich in omega 6 poly unsaturated fatty acids, generate aldehydes freely. Aldehydes promote cancer, heart disease - including associated hypertension and dementia. In fact, the World Health Organisation found that aldehyde levels, in these oils, were found to be twenty times higher than the recommended levels.

Are poly unsaturated fatty acids responsible for the chronic inflammation found in conditions like hypertension and associated conditions? It is quite possible given that arachidonic acid is a PUFA and that its end product is a leukotriene (LTB4) that has been found to be responsible for the chronic inflammation found in lymphoedema.

Studies have also shown that desaturase enzyme levels were elevated in many other chronic conditions including hypertension. Exactly what are desaturase enzymes?

These enzymes can convert fatty acids to either pro inflammatory or anti-inflammatory products. Inflammation helps us repair and heal by bringing much needed substances to the site of damage. At times of injury or illness pro inflammatory substances are required. However, when healing has taken place then the conversion of fatty acids to anti-inflammatory products is the desired outcome, otherwise chronic inflammation could be the consequence. However, desaturase enzymes require a number of other essential nutrients in order to respond appropriately to the body's status and avoid a state of chronic inflammation.

Over the years I have noticed that people whose diets are high in omega 6 PUFA's do have lined, unhealthy looking skin. Those who use saturated fats have healthy, well -nourished and unlined skin.

The Omega 3 'good' polyunsaturated fatty acids

Thankfully, there are some healthy oils although due to their reactive nature they are always better kept in a cool dark place and used as quickly as possible.

They benefit by reducing inflammation and come in three forms.

ALA – Alpha linolenic acid

EPA – Eicosapentaenoic acid

DHA – Docosahexanoic acid

Alpha linolenic acid is found mainly in plant oils such as flax seed and soy bean oil. It is an essential fatty acid which means that the body cannot make it and it has to be obtained from food sources. ALA can be converted to DHA and EPA but only in limited amounts.

DHA and EPA are found in animal sources, mainly oily fish and seafood. Most people do not eat enough oily fish to keep inflammation in check since the intake of the pro-inflammatory omega 6 fatty acids is, on average, six times higher than the levels of omega three fatty acids. In reality, it should be the other way around.

For those people who do not eat oily fish on a regular basis, supplementation with DHA and EPA is essential.

Table of food sources of Omega 3 – vegetarian and animal sources

Food	Type of Omega 3
salmon	DHA, EPA
oysters	DHA, EPA, ALA
sardines	DHA, EPA
trout	DHA, EPA
mackerel	
seaweed and algae	ALA, DHA, EPA
hemp seeds	ALA
flax seeds	ALA
walnuts	ALA
edamame	ALA
soybean	ALA
kidney bean	ALA
chia seeds	ALA
Brussel sprouts	ALA
kale	ALA
spinach	ALA

broccoli	ALA
cauliflower	ALA
chard	ALA

Monounsaturated fatty acids, the Dash diet compared to the Atkins diet

Monounsaturated fatty acids are also healthy fats found in some nuts, avocados and olive oil.

The Dash diet uses olive oil liberally along with recommendations for plenty of salad ingredients. It has been found to lower blood pressure and said to extend longevity. However, this diet will not work for everyone. Not everyone is a fan of olive oil nor can they cope with numerous foods of plant origin.

In some people it can help with weight loss, decrease inflammation and the risk of hypertension and cardiovascular disease but diets like the Atkins Diet have also had this effect.

The Atkins diet helps prevent the increase of blood sugars which triggers a release of insulin. Insulin is required to store fat in the form of triglycerides so anything which prevents this release will help reduce inflammation, help with weight reduction and prevent heart disease.

Fruit, as has already been explained, in spite of all the hyped health benefits has the potential to raise blood sugar levels dramatically.

In the end, if you are a fruit and vegetable lover and suffer no side effects from lectins or saponins then something similar to the Dash diet would be fine for you.

High fibre diets – containing lots of fruit and vegetables and whole grain products can be problematical for some people with irritable bowel syndrome or slow gut transit. Some people just like the taste of meat and therefore would be better sticking to a meat based diet although highly processed meat with lots of added salt should be avoided.

Salt is inflammatory in nature.

Sodium is implicated in triggering inflammatory disease as well as exacerbation and progression of the disease.

A study[8] showed high salt diets disrupt T cells and cause increased inflammation. This is something we should be

---

[8] https://www.nature.com/articles/s41590-018-0236-6

trying to avoid at all costs. Inflammation contributes to hypertension

Although we do excrete excess salt, it is thought that some may remain in micro-domains – small regions in the cell membrane. Some people are salt sensitive but, if this is the case it will have been picked up on the blood tests looking at the amount of renin and aldosterone in your system.

There are genetic differences in the way that excess sodium is dealt with in the body.

Some individuals appear to excrete excess sodium quite quickly but others may retain fluid and feel bloated.

More and more research has been undertaken on the impact of sodium. The findings have been along similar lines.

This is when taurine comes into its own. Taurine is an amino acid which is found in meat and fish although the latter has far higher levels of this substance. It is also added to some energy drinks.

Taurine acts as a natural diuretic keeping magnesium and potassium in the cells and sodium out of them.

This also includes any sodium in the micro-domains which could cause inflammation in the brain.

It also regulates calcium in certain cells, helps synthesise bile salts which help with fat digestion and supports the development of the nervous system.

It can be bought at good health food shops or online. It can be found in capsules, tablets or as a crystalline powder.

There are other useful amino acids for hypertension and we shall look at these later. You will find that most of them are in foods which are of animal origin. This may come as a surprise to many people that have been informed that the only healthy diet is one that relies heavily on fruit and vegetables.

Of course, it would be better if salt could be kept down to a minimum in the diet but we have been conditioned to like salt in foods and changes cannot always be made overnight no matter how sensible it may be to do so.

There are potassium based salts like Lo Salt. I have had mixed reviews on these. Some people swear that they cannot taste the difference and others use it once and say they never will again.

On a low salt diet, it is recommended that you eat less than 2000mg or 2gm of salt per day.

The Low sodium diet

The story goes that most people eat on average 5 teaspoons of salt per day which is approximately 20 times more than your body needs. The body needs only one quarter of one teaspoon daily and this does not need to be added salt. There is more than enough salt in the foods that you eat on a daily basis.

The processing and preparation of food generally includes sodium. For example, the raising agent used in scones and cakes contains good amounts of sodium.

One scone contains a quarter of your daily allowance of sodium, for example.

A pack of Hula Hoops contains half your daily allowance.

It's a good habit to get into looking at the information of processed food and convenience foods to see how much sodium they contain. Low sodium is defined as less than 140mg per serving. More than 400mg per serving is classed as being high in sodium.

Anything in brine or containing monosodium glutamate will automatically be high in sodium. Other foods to avoid are:

- Cured
- Smoked
- Canned meat or fish
- Sausage
- Salted nuts

Soft cheeses such as cottage cheese

   Spreads and sauces

   Prepacked vegetable juices

are some among many.

In addition, there are many medications that contain sodium such as

   Sodium Picosulphate

   Alka Seltzer

Food naturally contains sodium and sodium does not need to be added but we have become used to the taste and manufacturers respond to this.

There are, of course other ways of flavouring food. Clever cooks will add:

   Garlic

   Ginger

   Pepper

   Spices

   Herbs

   Citrus fruit

vinegar

Take too much sodium without adequate potassium and magnesium and lower extremities will begin to swell.

A useful guide to the amount of sodium in food can be found on www.calorieking.com.

At the end of this long chapter, it would be useful to recap on what has been learned.

Non-potassium sparing diuretics remove potassium, magnesium and zinc from the system as allegedly excessive fluid is removed.

The half-life of popular diuretics is short and the feedback system effective. Lost fluid will be replaced quickly due to increased thirst.

Diets are far too high in sodium (found in salted products) and too low in potassium and magnesium. This leads to swelling and high blood pressure.

Taurine found in meat and fish acts as a mild diuretic and helps to reduce blood pressure. However, some fish is high in sodium.

Diets high in fruit and vegetables do not necessarily lower blood pressure. They can cause high blood pressure through a number of mechanisms including preventing nitric oxide (a vessel dilator) from functioning.

An animal based protein diet can be healthier for some people than a mainly plant based diet. Diets along the Atkins type diet can lower cholesterol, initiate weight loss, lower blood pressure and help retain muscle mass (which also helps with weight loss).

Saturated fats are not responsible for inflammation. It is the 'healthy' vegetable oils that cause inflammation as they are unsaturated and have the potential to damage tissues including arteries.

Salt is inflammatory in nature. It is not necessary for health to be added to food as food naturally contains its own sodium.

Saturated fat does not raise blood sugar levels and therefore does not signal to the pancreas to release more insulin. Excess calories cannot therefore be stored as triglycerides as insulin is required for this process to occur.

Alpha blockers and all that

Alpha blockers are regularly prescribed for patients with high blood pressure. The most common one appears to be Doxazosin which has a frighteningly long list of side effects. Some of these include:

    Vertigo

    Headaches

    Swelling of feet and ankles or fingers

    Sudden urge to   pee

    Pain in lower abdomen

What do alpha blockers do?

Alpha blockers lower blood pressure by preventing a hormone – norepinephrine - from constricting the muscles in the walls of smaller vessels. Blood flow is improved and the relaxation of the blood vessels lowers blood pressure.

However, their main function is not to lower blood pressure. It is generally useful if you have an enlarged prostate. Doxazosin is generally taken for life although it is not generally recommended for elderly (that is, people over the age of 55 years).

Foods promoting nitric oxide which helps dilate vessel walls is preferable to taking alpha blockers, if possible.

These include:

Beets

Foods containing co enzyme Q10 as it helps preserve nitric oxide

Citrus fruits

Dark chocolate

Meat

Leafy green vegetables

Garlic

Nuts and seeds

The amino acid arginine and all foods containing this building block of protein

Arginine

Arginine is a non-essential amino acid which means that it is normally made within the body if the conditions are right. This may be harder to achieve as you age and metabolic processes become more inefficient.

Arginine changes into nitric oxide. Arginine is required to regulate blood flow and is often used in conditions where there is poor blood circulation. This includes:

Angina

Peripheral arterial disease

Erectile dysfunction

Pre-eclampsia

Intermittent claudication

as well as hypertension. In fact, if you have some of the above conditions as well as hypertension then it is a good sign that this is one area that needs addressing through changes to your diet.

In addition, arginine aids in:

- Wound healing
- Helping kidneys remove waste products from the body
- Helps maintain the immune system
- Arginine is found mainly in animal sources of protein such as fish, eggs and red meat.

Calcium channel blockers

Calcium channel blockers are often prescribed for those with high blood pressure. The most commonly prescribed is Amlodipine and it too, helps lower blood pressure by widening blood vessels.

It does this by inhibiting the influx of calcium ions across vascular smooth and cardiac muscle.

Amlodipine has a number of concerning side effects one of which is weakening of the lower limb muscles but many medications given for hypertension are also responsible for arrhythmias.

In addition, some other common symptoms include:

- Swelling
- Pulmonary oedema
- Flushing
- Nausea

Vertigo

Fatigue

palpitations

The best calcium channel blocker is magnesium. We have already looked at magnesium and magnesium rich foods and do not need to do so again.

In addition, the foods that can be substituted instead of alpha blockers are also true of calcium channel blockers.

ACE inhibitors nearly always figure in treatment for hypertension so the part on this type of medication is a little longer and more involved. There is some chemistry involved and some people will like this challenge and others not. If you are one of the latter, just pass it by and go onto the foods which can replace ACE inhibitors. It is not necessary for you to know how something works for it to work.

Angiotensin Converting Enzymes (ACE) (this part is taken from the book The Metabolic Syndrome Diet by Lynne D M Noble)

There are many different metabolic pathways responsible for blood pressure regulation by means of Angiotensin Converting Enzymes (ACE). They are related to the following systems

> Renin-angiotensin (RAS) also known as the renin-angiotensin-aldosterone system
>
> Renin-chymase (RCS)
>
> Kinin-nitric oxide (KNOS)
>
> Neutral endopeptide (NEPS)
>
> The one we have already looked at in some detail is the RAS system.

There are many food-originating ACE inhibitors which include antihypertensive peptides.

Ace inhibitors derived from food proteins are the best known group of bioactive peptides

Dairy foods are excellent ACE Inhibitors.

They treat **primary hypertension** very well indeed.

Primary hypertension occurs due to life style factors like obesity and lack of exercise.

If you are not obese and take regular exercise, then this chapter may not have as much relevance for you. However, if you are obese and fell running does not appeal to you, then this chapter may be relevant to you.

Secondary hypertension occurs due other medical conditions like kidney disease.

Antihypertensive peptides differ slightly at each end.

At one end is attached an amine group and this is called the N-terminal.

The amino acid residue on the other end has a carboxylic acid group attached to it and this is referred to as the C-terminal

Thus for simplicity

N------ | peptide | ———— C

There are specific amino acids residues which are typical for the N or C end of a peptide

The hydrophobic amino acids are characteristic of the N- end of a peptide and are specifically:

    Glycine

    Isoleucine

    Leucine

    valine

At the C end they are normally amino acids that are cyclic or have aromatic rings.

They comprise:

    proline

    tyrosine

    tryptophan

We can make good use of this knowledge for it now means that foods containing the above amino acids inhibit ACE thus preventing a rise in blood pressure.

It might be better to tabulate the different amino acids and look at good sources in food.

Table showing N terminal amino acids and their food sources

Amino acid residue	Food sources
Isoleucine	Beef chicken pork fish dairy beans lentil legumes whole grains seeds cocoa dark chocolate
Leucine	Chicken beef pork fish tofu canned beans milk cheese squash seeds and eggs
valine	beef chicken pork fish tofu yogurt beans podded peas seeds nuts and whole grains
glycine	any gelatinous compounds like gelatine, bone broth, organ meats meat with the skin or crackling left on

Table showing C terminal amino acids and their food sources

Amino acid residue	Food sources
Proline	Gelatin, chicken skin pork crackling proline milk soy protein
Tyrosine	Beef pork fish chicken tofu milk cheese beans seeds nuts and whole grains bananas
Tryptophan	Nuts seeds tofu cheese red meat chicken turkey fish oats beans lentil and eggs bananas

You will see that some of these foods are ones we have been told to avoid because they are bad for us such as pork crackling. I do not agree that pork crackling is bad for you in moderation.

For further foods that contain these amino acids. Nutrition data website can provide information.

These foods all contain ACE inhibitors and should be eaten on a daily basis for those with primary hypertension.

For chocolate lovers who are feeling left out, chocolate also contains the amino acid phenylalanine. This has an association with tyrosine – one of our C-terminal amino acid residues.

Phenylalanine is involved in making dopamine which is a brain chemical that can regulate mood.

It helps to stimulate the metabolism firing up the processes that give life

You will note that the tables do not include simple carbohydrates purely because simple carbohydrates do not contain the amino acids that we require to inhibit ACE that narrows blood vessels.

At the end of this long passage on foods that can replace blood pressure medications, we have learned some chemistry.

This stands us in good stead in understanding some of the many complex processes that underlie the mechanisms involving high blood pressure.

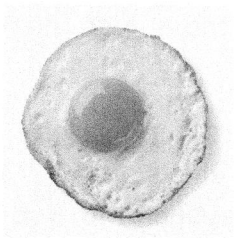

Eggs are a good source of N terminal amino acids

Blood thinners and anticoagulants

Blood thinners and anticoagulants are widely prescribed for people with hypertension because their condition is often associated with metabolic syndrome which encompasses a number of concerning medical concerns.

Rivaroxaban is a commonly prescribed blood thinner which has largely replaced Warfarin.

Rivaroxaban is a blood thinner or anticoagulant

It is taken if people have coronary heart disease or peripheral arterial disease among others.

Both of these conditions are associated with metabolic syndrome.

Side effects of this medication include:

    bleeding in the brain

- seizures
- changes to eyesight
- numbness or tingling
- tiredness, weakness
- feeling sick

there are a number of foods that are natural blood thinners and these include:

- turmeric
- ginger
- cinnamon (also lowers blood pressure)
- cayenne peppers
- vitamin E

WHOLE GRAINS

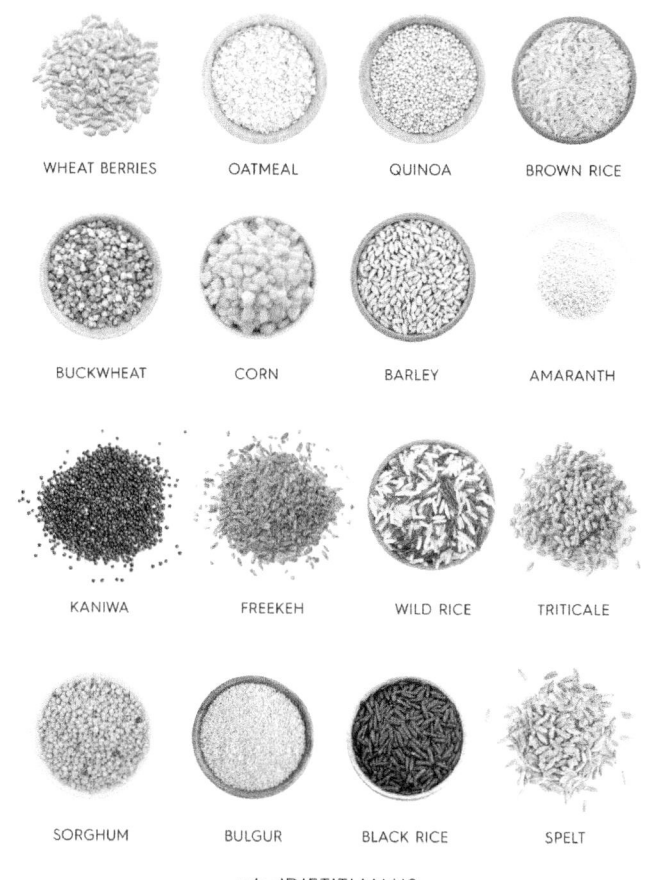

WHEAT BERRIES	OATMEAL	QUINOA	BROWN RICE
BUCKWHEAT	CORN	BARLEY	AMARANTH
KANIWA	FREEKEH	WILD RICE	TRITICALE
SORGHUM	BULGUR	BLACK RICE	SPELT

rebelDIETITIAN.US

Vitamin E is found in nuts, wheat germ, nut oils and whole grain foods.

These can be eaten without the side effects that many prescribed medications bring with them.

What if I am already on prescribed medications?

If you already on prescribed medications, then clearly you cannot stop them overnight. You may get a rebound action so that your blood pressure temporarily jumps up if a medication is stopped.

Initially, you need to implement the diet that helps to reduce your body mass and blood pressure.

It is helpful if measurements for these and waist circumference are logged.

After a couple of weeks compare the measurements again.

They should all have improved.

Continue for another couple of weeks.

Compare your results

As your body mass and blood pressure reduces. Your medication could be reduced.

This is because when medication is first prescribed it is partly based on your symptoms and your body mass.

It may be that if your blood pressure was very high initially you may have been placed on an ACE inhibitor and a diuretic.

One of these may now need to be withdrawn or at least a lower dose prescribed.

These reductions should be logged for they are great motivators when looking at the progress that has been made.

You will need to continue like this until you are not dependent on prescription medications to respond to conditions which are amenable to diet or, at the very least reduced them considerably.

Already, we have covered a lot of ground in looking how food can be our medicine.

Some people will no doubt enjoy putting together recipes that address the many issues of metabolic syndrome and associated hypertension.

Others will struggle either because they do not have cooking skills, the will or motivation or the time.

This will then take a little more planning because the emphasis here is creating your own dishes from scratch.

The other difficulty that people may have is the concept, for example, that chocolate is bad and fruit is good for you. We have been so conditioned to believe that many foods are bad for you when indeed they are not. The converse is also true.

I can only reiterate that chocolate - which is very high in cocoa solids - is an excellent food and eating fruit can lead to weight gain.

When nutritionists have extolled the virtues of fruit it is generally in terms of antioxidants and the amount of vitamin C fruit may contain.

It might be useful to recap antioxidant minerals and vitamins

These are:

Vitamins – E, C and beta carotene (carotene is found in orange coloured fruit and vegetables like carrots and pumpkin.

Minerals – copper, manganese, selenium and zinc

They all help to protect the body from free radicals which cause damage and inflammation in the body.

Selenium for example is used to make glutathione peroxidase which neutralises hydrogen peroxide in the body.

The best source of selenium is found in Brazil nuts.

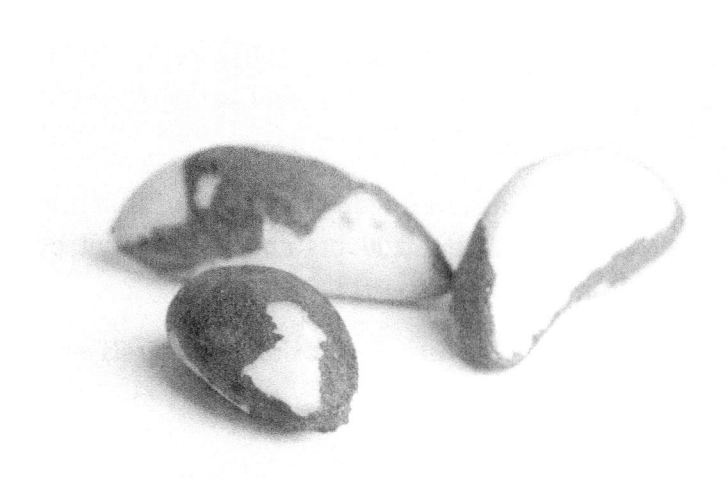

Two Brazil nuts provide all the recommended daily intake of selenium.

Angiotensin -2 receptor blockers (also known as ARB's)

These medications tend to end in 'sarten' such as Irbesartan which is one that is commonly prescribed. ARB's are useful in that they help prevent damage to the kidneys due to diabetes.

Like many other medications for high blood pressure they lower blood pressure by widening blood vessels.

Their action blocks angiotensin, a substance which narrows blood vessels.

However, the side effects of ARB's carry a long list. These include:

- sexual dysfunction
- chest pain
- musculoskeletal pain
- indigestion
- liver problems
- increased heartbeat
- hypersensitivity
- vasculitis
- muscle cramps
- altered taste

tinnitus

Natural ARB's are plentiful and include:

> potassium – you can see that if you take diuretics that a natural ARB may be in short supply

> Taurine

> Fibre

> Celery

> Co-enzyme Q10

> Vitamin B6 (Pyroxidone)

> Vitamin C

> Garlic

> Resveratrol

> Omega 3 fatty acids

Pyroxidone is one of the B complex vitamins.

Good sources of this vitamin are:

> Pork

> Poultry

> Oats

> Wheat germ

Peanuts

Soya beans

Bananas

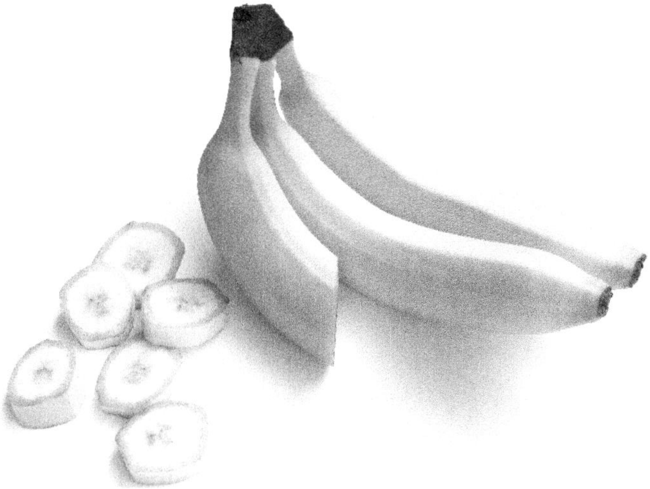

Bananas are a great source of Pyroxidone, potassium and fibre and are able to contribute to the maintenance of normal blood pressure.

Beta blockers

Beta blockers work by slowing down the heart by blocking noradrenaline. You will be aware of noradrenaline's actions if you have a fright for your heart will jump and your heart beat speed up.

Beta blockers are not for everyone with high blood pressure especially if you have a slow heart beat but they are useful for some people although they are not the first medication of choice for hypertension, normally. They are usually used as an adjunctive medication.

In addition, they are contraindicated in patients with:

Asthma or other lung diseases

Some circulatory problems such as Raynaud's syndrome where the extremities turn white or blue.

A prior allergic reaction to beta blockers

A condition known as metabolic acidosis

Patients taking medications for diabetes since beta blockers may hide the warning signs of low blood sugar.

Of course, since we are trying to block noradrenaline then medicines containing this or with similar action should be avoided. Many medications for allergies will contain these substances and should be avoided.

Some of these medications can be bought over the counter so if you suffer from allergies then it is better to discuss allergy medications with the pharmacist or your GP before purchasing.

Non-steroidal anti-inflammatory drugs (NSAID's) also have the capacity to increase blood pressure so NSAID's should be avoided for pain relief. There are plenty of other medications with analgesic properties and some nutritional supplements such as magnesium also have the capacity to reduce pain.

Like other medications used to control high blood pressure, beta blockers come with side effects. Not everyone suffers with them and, if they do, generally not all of them. The more common ones are:

Fatigue or light headedness (often symptomatic of a slower heart rate.

Insomnia and once asleep, nightmares.

Nausea

Compromised circulation to extremities leading to cold hands and feet

Urgent attention has to be paid to these side effects:

Wheezing, breathlessness, a tight feeling in the chest

Irregular heartbeat

Difficulty exercising or exercise is accompanied by a cough

Swollen ankles or legs

Jaundice like symptoms

Food alternatives to beta blockers

Fortunately, there are food sources which act as gentle alternatives to beta blockers. Many you will have met before.

These include:

Hawthorne. There are Hawthorne teas available in health food shops and some people make Hawthorne jelly as an accompaniment to meat.

Bananas – they block epinephrine and norepinephrine from attaching to the beta receptors

Omega 3 poly unsaturated fatty acids which we have already discussed.

Co-enzyme Q10

Niacin – vitamin B3

Magnesium

Niacin is found in:

Beef liver

Chicken or turkey breast

Salmon

Tuna

Pork tenderloin

Lentils

Banana

Peanuts

Brown rice

Fortified breakfast cereals

Amino acids as beta blockers

There are also a number of amino acids that act as beta blockers. Amino acids are the building blocks of protein. There are hundreds of different combinations of amino acids which produce different proteins. Thus the protein which forms connective tissue is very different from the protein which forms your hair.

Amino acids can be used therapeutically once you understand what properties they have. They are very affective in ameliorating common - and not so common – conditions.

We have come across some of these amino acids already. However, it would be helpful if they were tabulated with some description of them.

Amino acids which act as beta blockers

Amino acid	description
Gamma Amino Butyric Acid (GABA)	It is an amino acid that is produced naturally in the brain and functions at a neurotransmitter in the brain and central nervous system. Significant reduction has been achieved with 80mg daily. It aids sleep, relaxation and lowers blood pressure. It is found in fermented foods, whole grains, soy beans, lentils, most types of beans, potato, berries and cocoa

Taurine	A useful non-essential amino acid found in animal foods such as meat and fish. It helps stimulate metabolism. It is used in the synthesis of bile which is the main way of breaking down cholesterol It slows the progression of atherosclerosis where the build-up of plaque contributes to high blood pressure by narrowing the lumen of the blood vessels that the blood flows through.

L-theanine	**One of my favourites!** L-theanine has only three sources
	    Green tea
	    Black tea
	    Some types of mushrooms
	It promotes relaxation without drowsiness but can as it reduces anxiety effectively then it also assists those people whose insomnia is due to

	anxiety. 200mg has been shown to slow resting heart rate so would not be suitable for those with very slow heart rates.
Arginine	A non-essential amino acid widely found in a variety of animal protein with turkey breast providing the most per weight. Arginine is known to dilate arteries thus lowering blood pressure.

Please note that zinc is essential for a proper functioning protein metabolism. Without zinc, amino acids simply cannot fulfil their function.

Further, zinc is required for the synthesis of hundreds of enzymes and macromolecules some of which are involved in the breakdown of fats and carbohydrates needed for energy,

As we have seen, those on diuretics are particularly susceptible to zinc deficiency since zinc is flushed away along with the diuretic effect.

Thus diuretics may contribute to hypertension by other pathways not previously discussed.

Good sources of zinc are shellfish, milk, meat, legumes.

People eating a predominantly plant based diet are likely to be zinc deficient due to the phytates holding onto zinc so that it is not available to the body.

The recommended daily allowance is:

9mg for adult females

11mg for adult males.

However, zinc in much higher amounts is used at times of infection without detriment. It has excellent antiviral properties.

Zinc is one of those supplements that I keep in the medicine box at all times.

Counteracting fat storage, sugar cravings and primary hypertension

Many nutrients combat the tendency to fat storage. One of these is glutamine.

Glutamine is a conditionally essential amino acid. This means that under normal conditions the body will produce all that it needs but under times of stress and illness, more needs to be taken in the diet.

It is the most abundant amino acid in the body and blood with major functions in the immune system and intestines.

Glutamine can be converted to glucose directly in the kidneys. This conversion does not affect insulin so it contributes to energy without affecting insulin induced fat storage.

Research has born this out. Supplementation with glutamine resulted in a loss of body fat in those with a high fat diet.

In addition, as glutamine can provide energy then sugar cravings are reduced.

The B vitamins fat burning and reducing primary hypertension

The B complex has a major part to play in fat burning as they stimulate the breakdown of fat in the body.

As primary hypertension is caused by obesity and/or lack of exercise then anything that contributes to weight reduction is a bonus.

These B vitamins help control metabolism:

    Vitamin B12 (cobalamin)

Vitamin B2 (riboflavin)

Vitamin B3 (niacin)

Vitamin B5 (pantothenic acid)

Vitamin B7 (biotin)

Vitamin B2 is particularly important due to its ability to convert fats, carbohydrates and fats to energy. However, B vitamins should always be taken as a complex and always in the presence of zinc.

The vitamin B complex is a water soluble group of vitamins and so quite easily destroyed by light and heat or long storage.

Vitamin B12 needs an acidic environment in order for it to be separated from its protein source. This probably is not particularly relevant when young but stomach acid does decline with age. As it does so, food is not digested properly leading to indigestion.

The inappropriate response to this is to reduce acidity even further through the use of over the counter or prescription drugs so that inability to digest nutrients properly, leads to further ill health.

Most of the B complex can be found in wholegrains and red meat.

Riboflavin sources are:
- Milk
- Eggs
- Fortified breakfast cereals
- Mushrooms
- yogurt

Vitamin B complex, as a supplement is readily available at most supermarkets, health food stores – both high street and online. It is sold quite cheaply in supermarkets and is just as good and adequate as some of the more expensive one that you will find in some stores.

Vitamin B complex do have mild diuretic properties and also support the immune system.

Vitamin B3 was used to lower cholesterol levels before statins came onto the market.

Cholesterol is often unfairly blamed for promoting high blood pressure. When plaque, from arteries has been analysed, it has been found to contain just 3% cholesterol but a whopping 50% of calcium.

Calcium can be a bit of a thug if not deposited in the correct place. It can contribute to pain and inflammation. If there is adequate vitamin D in the diet, then calcium will be deposited in the bones rather than in arterial walls.

Cholesterol is a healing substance. It is required for the synthesis and maintenance of every cell in the body. It reduces inflammation, helps the skin absorb vitamin D from the sun's rays, helps form bile, boosts the immune system and neutralises bacterial toxins – just to mention a few of the hundreds of benefits that is has.

As people age, those with higher cholesterol levels have been found to live longer. They are less susceptible to infection, their skin is less thin and wrinkled. Cholesterol also contributes to the health of the brain where a large part of the brain and central nervous system is composed of cholesterol.

Statins prevent the synthesis of co-enzyme Q 10 which is a vital enzyme which helps lower blood pressure.

Niacin works to keep cholesterol to normal levels. At prescription level doses it helps to lower triglyceride levels and increase high density lipoprotein, reputedly the good cholesterol. It works simply by blocking the enzyme which aids the synthesis of cholesterol in the liver.

The recommended daily intake of niacin is:

16mg for adult males

14 mg for adult females

18mg during pregnancy

In cases of high cholesterol then doses of 500mg are given. However, this should be undertaken with

> **Food sources of niacin**
>
> **Chicken, turkey, beef and fish are the best sources. Legumes and nuts also provide some.**

Supervision as high doses of niacin can damage kidneys and the stomach lining.

Tryptophan – an amino acid – forms niacin. Tryptophan is found in milk, cheese, turkey and chicken breast, oats and canned tuna

However, consideration has to be given to what is thought to be high cholesterol. The idea that LDL is 'bad cholesterol' also needs to be reconsidered since it is this type that is associated with better memories and longevity. Indeed, one of the known side effects of taking statins is memory loss and it is the low density lipoprotein level that is being lowered through the use of statins.

Cholesterol naturally rises and falls with the demands of life place on it. Eat a high fat meal and cholesterol levels will rise because they are part of the composition of bile which is a substance needed to help with the digestion of fats.

If you have an infection them cholesterol levels will rise in order to help produce more immune system cells or neutralise bacterial toxins.

If you have injured yourself then cholesterol levels will rise because cells will need to be repaired or new ones formed.

Cholesterol is required for the synthesis of all hormones so if you artificially lower it you may find that you do not have optimum levels of vital hormones – the messengers in your system that tell your organs and tissues what to do at any given point.

The main indicator of stroke and heart disease is your blood pressure.

Of course, there are a few people who have greatly elevated levels of cholesterol – a condition known as hypercholesterolemia – which is often familial. However, this is present from birth and is often accompanied by

> tendon xanthomata which are hard, non-tender nodular enlargements of tendons. They are generally found on the knuckles of the hands

although they may occur on other tendons such as the Achilles tendon.

Xanthelasmata – small white lumps on the eyelids or face may also be symptomatic but I have known people with quite a cluster of these yet cholesterol tests have shown very low cholesterol levels so it is not an exact science.

Premature corneal arcus may also occur. Corneal arcus is the creamy coloured ring that surrounds the iris and is generally seen in some older people. I have known many older people in their late eighties with corneal arcus, who are fit, active, not taking statins and have a lively enquiring mind and no cardiovascular problems.

While doctors prefer to keep cholesterol levels under five, studies – on women at least – have shown that a cholesterol level of 7mmol is the optimum.

Sometimes non-familial hypercholesterolemia is considered to be present from 7.5mmol but the expectation is that some of the other signs already mentioned would be present.

Familial hypercholesterolemia is considered to be present when a level of 11mmol is reached.

You can see now that nothing is clear cut and while statins are often given as a 'preventative' it is the presence of high blood pressure that is the main indicator of cardiovascular events

If your cholesterol levels are only slightly raised, then it does not appear judicious to take statins given that cholesterol levels are dynamic and reducing levels may relieve you of the numerous benefits of cholesterol.

Arteriosclerosis and atherosclerosis

Arteriosclerosis and atherosclerosis both contribute to high blood pressure. They may be present together or just one may be present.

Arteriosclerosis is commonly referred to as 'hardening of the arteries.' It is an abnormal hardening of the arterial tissue where the arteries become less elastic providing resistance to blood flow.

The watch word is 'abnormal'. Many people dismiss arteriosclerosis as something that they would have to put up with as part of the ageing process. However, not everyone gets arteriosclerosis as they age so it is definitely not part of the ageing process.

In fact, most conditions that manifest themselves are not the result of genes. Yes, there may be a genetic propensity to certain conditions but genes can turn themselves on and off all the time due to prevailing environmental conditions.

While diet will not change your basic inherited genome, your genome does not have the final say in whether you will suffer from any condition. It is the **epigenome** that produces proteins and other molecules and it is these that regulate the genes by turning them on or off on the strands of DNA.

They are influenced by environmental factors, one of the greatest of which is nutritional substances.

If this were not so, why would health professionals encourage you to look at changing aspects of your diet.

However, the advice given by health professional can be restrictive and general when in fact it should be tailored to the individual. Animal based diets such as the Atkins Diet are not generally recommended although this diet can offer a great deal for someone suffering from hypertension.

Antioxidants are generally only seen as the domain of plants when actually some of the most effective antioxidants are seen in non-processed meat and other animal products.

So, back to arteriosclerosis. What will help keep your tissues supple and how do you know if arteriosclerosis may be a problem?

Nutrients for supple tissue

Vitamin C

Silica

Glycine

Vitamin D and vitamin K

We will look at these in turn.

Vitamin C

Vitamin C is a major player in the synthesis of connective tissue helping to promote proper formation. It also has excellent anti-inflammatory effects.

It is water soluble vitamin which is easily destroyed by heat and sunlight so good storage of vitamin C containing foods is a priority.

The RDA of vitamin C is set at a measly 30mg. This is far too low by anyone's standards. It is a level that was set to prevent scurvy but that's all. Much higher amounts are required for the many functions in the body. For example, research has shown that between 6000-8000mg daily will treat pneumonia as effectively as antibiotics.

Environmental stresses will also increase your need for vitamin C. Therefore, insomnia, pain, heat, illness will always increase the levels that you need to keep healthy and this will change on a day to day basis.

As it is impossible to determine individually how much to prescribe patients we use something called bowel tolerance as a guide. Simply, when you have taken in enough vitamin C for your body's need it will result in loose bowels.

On one day you may find that 1000mg may be enough and on the next day your need for vitamin C rises to 3000mg.

In addition, if you are a smoker then for every cigarette smoked, 30mg of vitamin c is used to neutralise the impact of the toxins in them. Smokers tend not to have very good diets in the first place and are unlikely to eat enough vitamin C in their diets, to cover this, never mind the rest of their body's needs.

The main sources of food are raw fruit and vegetables. Lightly cooked they will lose some of their vitamin C. One orange contains 30mg so if you do have an infection or inflammatory condition, it takes a lot of fruit and vegetables to reach optimum levels.

If you are one of those people who don't eat many fruit or veg – for whatever reason – then supplementing with vitamin C would not come amiss. In addition, vitamin C supplements are useful to have in the medicine cabinet since large doses (6-8g) have been found to have a therapeutic effect against bacterial pneumonia.

Silica

Silica is a natural substance which can be found in the planet's crust. Indeed, one quarter of it makes up the sands, rocks and clay that are part of our environment.

There has been some research that has shown that silica helps form the building blocks of collagen. Collagen is a protein which forms a major part of the many types of connective tissue that you have in your body.

Collagen keeps the skin supple and elastic. It prevents wrinkling. As the arteries are also formed from collagen then attention to good collagen formation is vital.

Good sources of silica are:

    oats

    cucumber

    wholegrain

    rice

    green beans

Glycine

A number of amino acids have been shown to prevent arterial stiffness but the one that stands out is glycine. Glycine is the smallest amino acid and non-essential in the sense that the body – if conditions are right – will synthesise it.

Glycine is a major component of collagen. Hypertension is a condition in which free radicals and large vessel elasticity contribute. Glycine assists in lowering blood pressure by reducing the generation of free radicals which assists in a reduction of arterial stiffness. However, as a major component of collagen and elastin, any deficiency of glycine would impair the formation of these critical connective tissues compromising the elasticity of the aorta.

Studies of those with metabolic syndrome have found that supplementation with glycine has led to a significant decrease in systolic blood pressure.

Before we look at the role of vitamin D and K it might be a good idea to introduce the concept of atherosclerosis.

Atherosclerosis is often mixed up with arteriosclerosis but whereas the latter is all about the stiffness of arteries, atherosclerosis describes the build-up of plaque inside the arteries.

The plaque is composed of cellular waste, fibrin, fats, calcium and cholesterol. As plaque builds up the diameter of the lumen of the artery becomes smaller. Blood flow is reduced. The heart is trying to pump blood through a much constricted vessel and, as such, the pressure is increased.

Bits of plaque can break off and get stuck in smaller vessels so that tissues are not oxygenated. When tissues die we refer to it as an infarction. Blood clots may develop in vessels which are no longer smooth and conducive to good blood flow.

Vitamin D and Vitamin K can be used to work against arterial stiffness and plaque formation and it only takes simple lifestyle changes to do this

Vitamin D and vitamin K

Healthy arteries are formed from 3 layers. The inner layer – the endothelium – is easily disrupted by:

> raised blood sugar levels

> inflammation

If inflammation or raised blood sugar levels occur, then the damage they inflict on delicate arteries increases the stiffness. As this increases blood pressure, the resulting increase in blood pressure begins to inflict further damage on these vessels.

The main cause is not cholesterol. The main factor that contributes to arteriosclerosis is calcium being abnormally deposited in artery wall. This is known as calcification and, as its name suggests, really does result in stiffening of the arteries.

Fortunately, the vitamins D and K can prevent this process from happening.

We have already ascertained that vitamin D is required to open the door for calcium to enter bones. Without sufficient vitamin D, calcium will be dumped anywhere including in the arteries. Calcium, in the wrong place is more than capable of damaging tissues and creating pain so anyone with hypertension needs to ask to have their vitamin D levels checked.

Vitamin D can be measured using either nmol/L or in ng/ml. Normally, in the UK they are measured in nmol/L. You don't have to know what these mean, just refer to the chart below for guidance.

It is unlikely that anyone is obtaining sufficient vitamin D through diet alone. The sun is the best source but we do not have many days when we can harness the sun's rays. Certainly, the days between the end of April and the end of September are the only ones likely to have enough sun to help synthesise vitamin D under the skin.

A poor summer, lack of sufficient cholesterol (vitamin D synthesis requires cholesterol) or ageing which impairs vitamin D synthesis or absorption in the gut all conspire to cause a deficiency of vitamin D.

Vitamin D3 is the active form if you choose to go down the route of supplementation. Vitamin D needs to be taken with a little fat for it to be absorbed. Those on low fat/no fat diets are likely to be deficient in fat soluble vitamins including vitamin D.

If you find that you are deficient in vitamin D, then supplement of 2000-4000Iu's should be taken. In any case, this would be a judicious strategy from the end of September until the beginning of May so that you benefit from this remarkable vitamin during the time of seasonal respiratory infections and lack of sunshine.

Table showing vitamin D status[9]

Vitamin D status	nmol/L	ng/mL
Optimal	100–150	40–60
Sufficient	75–99	30–39
Insufficient	50–74	20–29
Deficient	<50	<20

Vitamin D tests can be obtained over the counter at pharmacists but check that the tests give you an indication of your level of vitamin D other than insufficient or sufficient. You really are aiming for optimal levels.

Vitamin K

Many people have heard of vitamin K but will have no idea what it does or which food sources it is obtained from. In fact, there are two forms of vitamin K with strange sounding names. These are:

phylloquinone (vitamin K1)

menoquinone (vitamin k2)

A higher intake of vitamin K2 is associated with a lower risk of cardiovascular disease but K1 is not.

---

[9] https://www.hindawi.com/journals/dm/2015/864370/

Vitamin K2 inhibits vascular calcification and like vitamin D also exerts anti-inflammatory effects. It blocks the progression of arterial thickening and stiffening and reduces the chance of dying from heart disease by nearly 60%.

In addition, as vitamin K2 activates proteins that keep calcium in bones and out of arteries, it has also been found to reduce non-vertebral fractures by 81%.

A study[10] looked at two groups.

Group 1 - received 90mcg of vitamin K daily plus 400 IU's of vitamin D

Group 2 – received 400 IU's of vitamin D daily.

It was fund that there was slower progress of the common carotid intima media thickness which is a good indicator of atherosclerosis.

How does vitamin K2 work to slow the progression of atherosclerosis? Well, vitamin K2 is required to activate a protein that keeps calcium in bones and out of arteries. In many respects it works along similar lines to vitamin D.

---

1. [10] Kurnatowska I, Grzelak P, Masajtis-Zagajewska A, et al. Effect of vitamin K2 on progression of atherosclerosis and vascular calcification in nondialyzed patients with chronic kidney disease stages 3-5. *Pol Arch Med Wewn*. 2015;125(9):631-40.

If I have any concerns regarding this study, it is the low dose of vitamin D used in the study. 400 IU's was originally set in the 1950's as the minimum dose required to prevent rickets. The recommended daily dose is really much higher so it is not surprising that there did not appear to be any therapeutic effect from 400 IU's.

In contrast, the recommended daily dose of vitamin K is 1mcg for every kilogram a person weighs. A study dose of 90mcg is likely to be the optimum dose for most people in that study.

People who have been on blood thinners like Warfarin (Coumadin) will have been advised to avoid foods containing vitamin K as this vitamin helps blood to clot. Warfarin blocks the action of vitamin K.

The idea of a blood thinner is to enable blood to flow more easily and prevent clots but blocking the action of vitamin K will result in a quicker build-up of plaque and resulting hypertension. Plaque can cause blockages, break off and lodge in smaller arteries causing the death of surrounding tissue through lack of oxygen to the tissues.

There are other blood thinners such as Rivaroxaban but there is no antidote to this medication. People do bleed to death. Burst blood capillaries – especially seen in the eyes – spontaneous bruising, peeing blood, among other symptoms are not unusual.

The test is your blood pressure. Take measures to reduce this and your need for blood thinners is also lowered.

If you suffer from bone problems such as osteoporosis or osteopenia – as well as hypertension - then you do need to consider increasing food sources of vitamins K and D. They may not look as though they have a common root deficiency but they do.

Vitamins D and K are both fat soluble vitamins and cannot be absorbed without a little fat in the diet. Therefore, those on low fat diets are at risk of deficiency of these two vitamins.

Vitamin K and elastin

Elastin is a type of connective tissue which provides that springiness to tissues. Sagging skin and wrinkly skin are probably deficient in good elastin.

Elastin contains Matrix Gla protein (MGP). A deficiency of vitamin k will lead to impaired MGP due to an increase of the calcium content within the elastin fibres.

When elastin calcification occurs it promotes the degradation of elastin. Elastin is vitally important to maintain supple blood vessels without which arteriosclerosis and resultant hypertension would occur.

Sources of vitamin K2

The best sources of vitamin K2 are:

    organ meats like liver, kidney and heart

    egg yolks

    cheese

    natto (fermented soya beans)

    most fermented dairy foods like yogurt

Unfortunately, patients are often advised to avoid foods like organ meats, egg and cheese as they are supposed to be bad for those with hypertension. Nothing is bad in moderation. Take cheese with adequate vitamin D and the calcium it contains will end up in bones where it was meant to be. Yes, eggs (and organ meats) contain cholesterol but they both have inbuilt vitamin B complex which more than adequately deals with any excess there may be.

In addition, take in too much dietary cholesterol and your amazing liver will adjust and make less until equilibrium is restored.

By now, I expect that some of this information may have caused your head to reel a little. There is far more to hypertension than just reducing salt and, in some cases, reducing salt in those who are not salt sensitive is not useful.

A diet rich in fruit and vegetables may cause hypertension in susceptible people and a meat based diet may be better in many cases. Fermented foods, like cheese, may be just the ticket for patients who need to include more vitamin K in their diet.

Diets low in good fats will deprive us of the ability to absorb fat soluble vitamins which are vitamins A, D, E and K. It is the fat soluble vitamins that have a major positive impact on hypertension and cardiovascular disease.

Your test results will give you an indication of what is causing your hypertension. This book will not just recommend one particular diet which cannot possible fit all but will help you address specific areas which are specific to you. In some cases, it may take only a couple of tweaks which is far easier to address than changing a diet whole scale.

Some causes of obesity

Obesity may or may not contribute to hypertension. Obesity is actually difficult to define because a measure known as the BMI (body mass index) is used. It would be helpful to take a look at why the BMI is not a good indicator of health.

The BMI Index is invalid

When people attend their General Practitioner then one of the measurements taken at the time is body mass. This is then plotted on a chart and the results are channelled into a bald statement which determine whether you are

Underweight

Normal weight

Obese

Morbidly Obese

The Body Mass Index (BMI) is not an accurate measure of fat. It doesn't explain the causes of poor health, either.

In some cases, obesity can be a risk factor for diabetes, heart disease and death but only in those with a genetic propensity to such illnesses.

In many cases obesity actually increases survival time in those with chronic illness. Therefore, individuals with a high BMI with chronic illness such as heart failure or kidney failure, among others, are more likely to have increased survival rates. It is thought that having more fat provides additional energy reserves.

The guidelines set by the World Health Organisation (WHO) stated that a BMI of over 25 is considered to be overweight while a BMI of more than 30 would indicate that the individual is obese. However, this criterion fails to take into consideration a number of groups for which such criterion would fail to apply.

The criterion fails to address large number of people in Asia such as Japanese and Koreans. They experienced metabolic risks, such as diabetes and hypertension, at a much lower threshold. Even with a BMI of 23 or 24, studies found that a significant number of people of Japanese or Korean descent had those diseases.

Studies also show that the current BMI recommendations are not suitable for older adults.

A study undertaken by Caryl Nowson, who was a professor of nutrition and aging at Deakin University, examined the relationship between BMI and risk of death in people 65 and over. The findings indicated that there was a lower risk of death in those with a BMI which fell into the obese category. Further, it was found that mortality increased significantly among those with a BMI in the 'normal' weight range. Further studies found that those with BMI in the obese range had a reduced risk of dying compared to those whose BMI was 21 or 22 – that is, in the normal range. The findings were that, 'by current standards, being overweight is not associated with an increased risk of dying.

Professor Nowson stated

Rather it is those sitting at the lower end of the normal range that need to be monitored, as older people with BMI's less than 23 are at an increased risk of dying.'

He added

Rather than focussing on weight loss, older people should put their efforts into having a balanced diet, eating when hungry and keeping active.'

Some studies have demonstrated that some obese individuals have a lower cardiovascular risk while many individuals with a normal BMI are metabolically unhealthy and have an increased mortality risk.

Obesity is not always associated with joint problems. Inflammation is generally associated with joint problems and this is more of a concern of nutritional intake rather than obesity. Of course with any medical condition some individuals have more of a propensity to such conditions, than others. That means they will have to pay more attention to their diets than those not predisposed to joint problems.[11]

Obese people have better post-surgical short-term survival rates among obese people than patients of 'normal' weight.' Patients with a BMI of 23.1 or less

---

[11] Glycine and phenylalanine, chondroitin and glucosamine are nutrients which assist in good joint health.

were more than twice as likely to die within 30 days of surgery than those with a BMI of 35.5 or more.

The BMI also exaggerates thinness in short people and fatness in tall people. Further, it does not take into account the person's body fat versus muscle (lean tissue). As such it is a very flawed measure of a person's body fat.

It is not worth the paper it is printed on since it was devised for an entirely different purpose.

However, if you feel that your hypertension may be related to your body mass then reducing your energy intake may be a good idea if you have ruled our other causes.

Unfortunately, there are many causes of higher body mass that do not include excess energy intake. Here are some of them.

Antibiotics

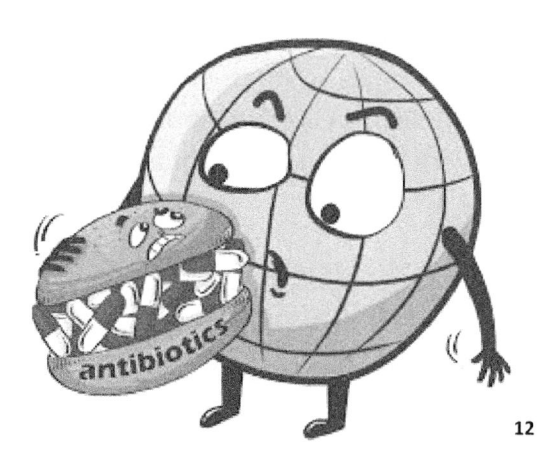

I've taken too many unnecessary antibiotics.

One of the unwanted side effects of antibiotics which tends not to reach the leaflets enclosed with the medication is that can produce significant weight gain.

Gut bacteria have numerous functions in your body and can play a role in obesity. Studies have shown that exposure to antibiotics in early life may have long term consequences for a child's metabolism.

Mice given antibiotics for the first four weeks of life grew up to be 25% heavier. They also had 60% more body fat than the controls.

---

[12] http://www.chinadaily.com.cn/opinion/2016-11/17/content_27401092.htm

Earlier research also showed that mice fed antibiotics – in doses similar to those given to children for throat or ear infections had significant increases in body fat despite their diets remaining unchanged.

There is an association between the composition of the intestinal microbiota and obesity. This has been demonstrated by studies showing differences in microbiota composition between obese and lean humans.

Obesity is associated with an increase of the phylum Firmucutes and a decrease in Bacteroidetes which are partly attributable to diet.

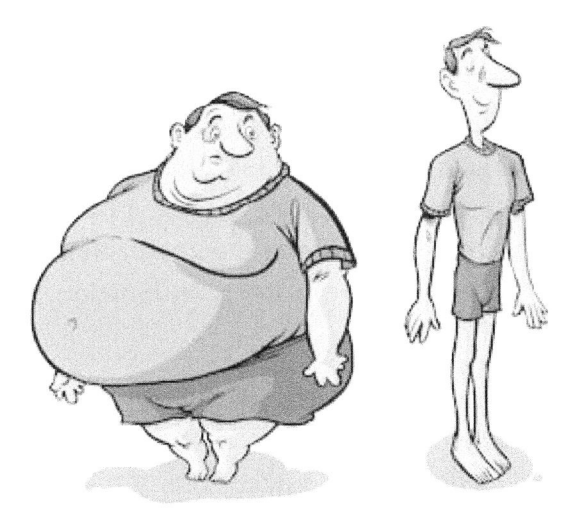

Left: microbiota of increased Firmucute. Right: microbiota of increased Bacteroidetes

When a low energy diet is taken then there is a shift in gut microbiota with a decrease in Firmucutes.

It has been found that this is similar to the gut bacteria found in a lean person.

When calorie intake is increased then Firmucutes multiplies reflecting the microbiota of obese people.

The judicious use of antibiotics is of paramount importance. Antibiotics do not work on many infectious agents such as viruses and unwise prescribing can lead to antibiotic resistance as well as obesity.

Alternative remedies for common ailments need to be explored. Further, we also need to look at how we can harness our own defences in order to avoid the overuse of antibiotics. Rest, moderate exercise and nutritionally sound meals help our immune systems to function as they should.

Attention should be paid to vitamin D3 and zinc intake in the colder months since they are vital nutrients in fighting infection. Further, adequate levels of vitamin D3 have been found to be associated with modest reductions in weight.

Stress

Whenever the body is under a state of stress, it releases cortisol. Cortisol is the anti-stress hormone and when it is released into the bloodstream it can act on many different parts of the body and help it to respond to stress or danger.

Cortisol also helps increase the body's metabolism of glucose.

Cortisol is a necessary stress hormone that is designed to

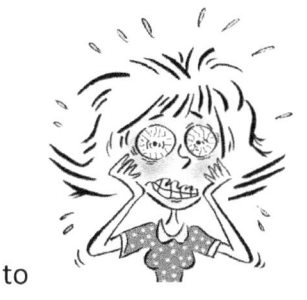

Stress can increase the risk for obesity

aid wakefulness in the mornings as well as enable us to cope with danger. An increase in cortisol also triggers the release of amino acids from the muscles, fatty acids into the blood stream as well as glucose from the liver.

This all helps us access an enormous amount of energy should we need it in an emergency.

Cortisol also stimulates insulin release and maintenance of blood sugar levels. The consequence of all the above is an increase in appetite especially in relation to sweet, high fat and salty foods.

Insulin resistance is a particular problem as it may lead to an increase in blood sugar. High blood sugar levels can cause a lot of systemic damage. We really want the blood sugar to be pushed into cells and provide fuel for cells rather than circulate in the blood. This is what provides our energy.

When insulin resistance abounds, weight gain is one of the side effects.

We can translate the effects of cortisol to other stressors in our life which have the potential to cause weight gain.

Often we have been so inculcated into thinking that our way of life is the 'norm' that we don't explore the damage that it is doing to us. Some common examples of stressors which have the potential to raise cortisol and impact weight are:

Caffeinated drinks

Lack of sleep

Driving

Light pollution

Noise pollution

Relationship difficulties

Working in a less than satisfying job

Not having enough time to do things

Being too cold

Being too hot

Children

Illness

Injury

Dealing with utilities and similar organisations

Divorce

Bereavement

Please feel free to add some of your own.

Insomnia is associated with obesity.

It is perhaps not difficult to see that the more developed our lives or countries are, the more likely we are to suffer from *unwanted* obesity that is not necessarily associated with over eating.

Extended exercise (more than 20 minutes) will use up the energy released by cortisol. It will also help to control insulin resistance so that the fuel released can be used by cells.

When cortisol levels are elevated, the body also produces less testosterone. This will result in a decrease in muscle mass. You need testosterone to build muscle mass.

Muscle helps to burn calories. However, a reduced muscle mass, will burn fewer calories.

Stress can also alter the normal pattern of cortisol secretion. Normally levels are highest in the morning and lowest at night. As levels of cortisol lessen, melatonin increases.

Melatonin is a hormone which regulates the sleep wake cycle. When melatonin is disrupted by wayward cortisol levels then sleep escapes us.

This disrupted sleep pattern causes further stress. A vicious circle begins.

This disruption of cortisol secretion doesn't just promote weight gain; it also decides where that weight gain will occur. Stress coupled with elevated cortisol will cause fat deposition in the abdominal area as opposed to the hips.

This apple shaped abdominal obesity is unhealthy, compared to the pear shaped figure of an obese individual, where such fat deposition has not been caused by raised cortisol levels.

It is the apple shaped abdominal fat deposition which is associated with cardiovascular disease which includes stroke and heart attacks. This is a far better indicator of poor health than the BMI.

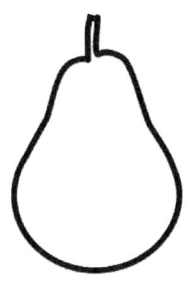

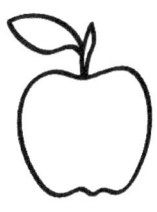

Better pear shaped than apple shaped.

If you find that you have a tendency to an apple shape, then you need to investigate the stressors in your life and seek to eliminate them. This isn't always easy and sometimes an innovative approach has to be considered, or help sought from other quarters. For example, if money is tight then

- growing your own food or
- learning how to harvest it for free from the countryside or

- joining a cookery class which teaches you how to cook cheaper meals, can help as well as provide new friendships.

Some people love living frugally – I do – but others find it stressful.

If coffee is a stressor, then find a decaffeinated blend or try something entirely different. I am not keen on herbal teas but I don't mind the decaffeinated black teas at all.

Symptoms of excessive cortisol levels are

> Weight gain around the upper back
>
> Rounding of the face
>
> Flushed face
>
> Thinning skin
>
> Easy bruising
>
> Muscle weakness
>
> Delayed healing

Exercise and the Lymphatic System

The lymphatic system runs parallel to the circulatory system. It contains hundreds of lymphatic vessels and bean shaped nodes throughout the body. It carries a clear fluid known as lymph throughout the body. This fluid helps to deliver essential white blood cells to sites of infection to fight disease

The lymph system can become clogged with dead bacteria and other waste. Unlike the circulatory system which has a pump – the heart – the lymphatic system does not. To get lymph moving you need to move. It is a slow process unclogging the lymphatic system but the consequences of this, if exercise is not undertaken, is that swelling will occur. If it is allowed to continue then infection and disease will occur.

When lymph builds up it can cause weight gain but this is due to lymph not adipose tissue.

It can also increase the need for a larger clothing size.

Lymph can be helped to move by **light** support.

Lymph has to travel against gravity so it has an uphill struggle. Tight clothing, however, does not help at all. The lymph vessels are very delicate and tight clothing will just compress them so that the lymph cannot flow. Therefore, when out walking, wear comfortable loose clothing.

Slow, relaxed breathing also helps to activate the lymph system. Our general pattern of breathing has become quicker and shallower and generally reflects the fast pace of life which is ours.

A considerable amount of weight can be lost without dieting just by attending to the needs to the lymphatic system. Dry brushing and elevating the foot of the bed is also beneficial for getting lymph to flow.

There is also a special form of light massage called lymphatic drainage which may be beneficial. However, the weight that will be lost will not be fat, it will be excess lymph fluid which can weigh a considerable amount. While fat is not lost, the excess fluid lost can result in a much more contoured shape.

A clogged lymphatic system is more likely in

> The elderly
>
> Those who have had a recent infection
>
> Those who don't exercise much
>
> Those who have had an injury which has damaged the fragile lymph vessels

Lymphoedema differs in that it is a chronic disease and requires much more and ongoing attention.

However, a poorly functioning or clogged lymphatic system can cause significant weight gain which has nothing to do with an excess of calories.

Some medications which cause weight gain

It is probably true to say that there are more medications which induce weight gain than there are which result in weight loss. Unfortunately, many of these are medications which are prescribed on a frequent basis.

Antihistamines are well known for causing significant weight gain. They appear to do this by inhibiting histamine. Histamine is released as an early response to injury or the presence of an allergen. It causes symptoms such as itchy, runny noses, urticaria (nettle rash) streaming eyes, among others. It can also cause achy joints and muscles in some people.

Histamine suppresses appetite so one effect of taking antihistamines is an increase in appetite. This doesn't appear to be the whole story, in our quest for causes of weight gain, since some antihistamines appear to cause more weight gain than others; currently. there does not appear to be a known explanation for this.

Studies have shown that those taking antihistamines can be up to two stone heavier than those who aren't.

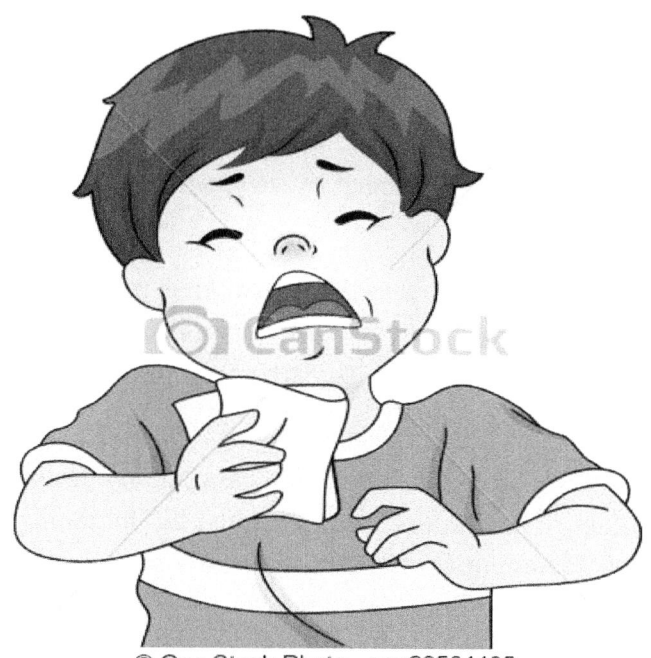

Anti-histamines are taken by people with allergies

Some high histamine foods are

　Pickled foods

　Fermented food such as sauerkraut, yogurt, sour cream, buttermilk, kefir, cheese

　Cured or fermented meats – sausages, salami and fermented ham.

If your diet is high in these foods it is quite likely that you will have unwanted weight gain if you are taking antihistamines to cope with the side effects of a high histamine diet.

The two main culprits of antihistamines are

>Fenofexadine

>Cetirizine

Antihistamines also have a sedating effect and it may account for less exercise being taken so that calorie expenditure is reduced.

This explanation cannot account for the whole story though. Some antacids such as Ranitidine and Omeprazole, which act on similar receptors, also cause quite marked weight gain and without the sedating effects. It may be that a reduction in symptoms which such antacids bring may increase a desire to eat. However, I am not sure that this accounts for the marked increase in weight gain that antihistamines and antacids bring. Ranitidine has been found to cause modest weight loss in some individuals too.[13]

---

[13] Ranitidine has also be found to cause modest weight loss in some people.

A natural substance, quercetin, which is found in many vegetables especially those in the onion family have been found to counteract allergies but without the side effects/weight gain of antihistamines.

Non-steroidal anti-inflammatory drugs (NSAID's)

NSAID's such as ibuprofen do not cause an increase in body fat, but they do cause weight gain in the form of excess water, known as oedema. As Ibuprofen will not increase your appetite, any weight gain, due to excess water, will disappear once the medication has been stopped.

NSAID'S should not be used in those with kidney problems or those on methotrexate. They are often implicated in allergies, or anaphylaxis, for which the treatment offered is an antihistamine.

As we have seen these have the potential to cause weight gain, oedema and consequently, high blood pressure.

Medication for neuropathic pain

Most medication for neuropathic pain such as that prescribed for those with MS has a reputation for piling on the pounds. The reasons for this have been attributed to their ability to increase appetite; they also have a tendency to cause oedema.

Pregabalin is also used for treating epilepsy, shingles pain, diabetic neuropathy and anxiety. This means that, as a whole, these types of medications, which are prescribed widely, are contributing to obesity.

Pregabalin works in a number of different ways

> It reduces the electrical activity which causes seizures in those with epilepsy.

> With nerve pain it blocks pain by interfering with the pain messages travelling from the brain to the spine.

> Pregabalin addresses anxiety by preventing your brain from releasing the chemicals that make you feel anxious.

Magnesium, a mineral which is involved in over 700 enzymatic actions in the body, is able to address all the above and may be used to replace Pregabalin and without the associated weight gain.

We have now finished our exploration of high blood pressure, the major underlying causes, the medications that may be prescribed and, just as importantly, how some of those medications can be replaced by making tweaks to diet.

We have seen that there is no one specific diet that will respond to everyone's needs. We have discovered that fruit sugar (fructose) may be the cause of high blood pressure and that diuretics, often prescribed for those with hypertension, may make this condition worse through the loss of important electrolytes during diuresis.

We have seen how stress may contribute to hypertension. While some stressors - such as the loss of a much loved partner - are not so easily addressed, many people find solace in walking, with a friend or alone, in the countryside. Simple measures like these can have a major role to play in reducing blood pressure.

When you have finished reading this book you should have a good idea of your own unique factors that have led to a diagnosis of hypertension and can take those first steps to reversing it.

Habberley Valley Visitor Centre and Tea Room

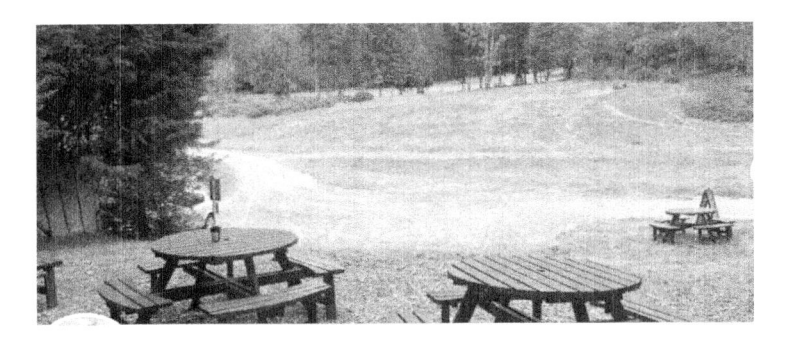

Walking in beautiful surroundings helps to lower blood pressure

Habberley Valley, approximately two miles north west of Kidderminster on the B4190 between Franche and Bewdley is an area of outstanding beauty in the district of Wyre Forest. It boasts one of the best heaths in Worcestershire, an ancient woodland and high sandstone cliffs.

The Habberley Valley Circular (yellow) route is approximately a 5km loop trail. It is rated moderately easy and due to the wild flowers is primarily used for nature trips as well as hiking.

Set in the heart of the valley, Steve and Wendy provide a friendly welcome in their family run tea room which overlooks this picturesque landscape.

Selling hot and cold drinks, cobs, sandwiches, Paninis and cakes and ice creams, the tea room has a 5- star hygiene rating.   Debit cards and cash are accepted.

We have found the prices to be the best, locally.

If you want to know about Habberley Valley's history, Steve is happy to provide that too. A unique set of mounted photo's takes you through its history.

The tea room is currently open from 10am-4pm from Wednesday to Sunday. These hours may be extended as summer approaches.

For more information, Steve and Wendy can be contacted on Facebook under

Habberley Valley Visitor Centre

You may find the book The Metabolic Syndrome Diet – by the same author - a useful companion to this book.

Printed in Great Britain
by Amazon